Body Shaping

Procedures in Cosmetic Dermatology
Series Editor: Jeffrey S. Dover MD FRCPC FRCP
Associate Editor: Murad Alam MD MSCI

Botulinum Toxin
Third edition
Alastair Carruthers MA BM BCh FRCPC FRCP and Jean Carruthers MD FRCSC FRC(Ophth) FASOPRS
ISBN 978-1-4557-2781-0

Soft Tissue Augmentation
Third edition
Jean Carruthers MD FRCSC FRC(Ophth) FASOPRS and Alastair Carruthers MA BM BCh FRCPC FRCP
ISBN 978-1-4557-2782-7

Cosmeceuticals
Third edition
Zoe Diana Draelos MD, Murad Alam MD MSCI and Jeffrey S. Dover MD FRCPC FRCP
ISBN 978-0-323-29869-8

Lasers and Lights
Third edition
George J. Hruza MD and Mathew Avram MD
ISBN 978-1-4557-2783-4

Treatment of Leg Veins
Second edition
Murad Alam MD and Sirunya Silapunt MD
ISBN 978-1-4377-0739-7

Photodynamic Therapy
Second edition
Mitchel P. Goldman MD
ISBN 978-1-4160-4211-2

Chemical Peels
Second edition
Rebecca C. Tung MD and Mark G. Rubin MD
ISBN 978-1-4377-1924-6

Non-Surgical Skin Tightening and Lifting
Murad Alam MD MSCI and Jeffrey S. Dover MD RCPC FRCP
ISBN 978-1-4160-5960-8

Scar Revision
Kenneth A. Arndt MD
ISBN 978-1-4160-3131-4

Hair Transplantation
Robert S. Haber MD and Dowling B. Stough MD
ISBN 978-1-4160-3104-8

Liposuction
C. William Hanke MD MPH FACP and Gerhard Sattler MD
ISBN 978-1-4160-2208-4

Body Contouring
Bruce E. Katz MD and Neil S. Sadick MD FAAD FAACS FACP FACPh
ISBN 978-1-4377-0739-7

Advanced Face Lifting
Ronald L. Moy MD and Edgar F. Fincher MD
ISBN 978-1-4160-2997-7

Blepharoplasty
Ronald L. Moy MD and Edgar F. Fincher MD
ISBN 978-1-4160-2996-0

PROCEDURES IN COSMETIC DERMATOLOGY

Body Shaping:
Skin • Fat • Cellulite

Edited by

Jeffrey Orringer MD
Professor and Chief, Division of Cosmetic Dermatology,
University of Michigan, Ann Arbor, MI, USA

Jeffrey S. Dover MD FRCPC FRCP
Associate Clinical Professor of Dermatology, Yale University School of Medicine;
Clinical Professor of Surgery, Dartmouth Medical School;
Adjunct Associate Professor of Dermatology, Brown Medical School;
Director, SkinCare Physicians, Chestnut Hill, MA, USA

Murad Alam MD MSCI
Professor of Dermatology, Otolaryngology, and Surgery;
Chief, Section of Cutaneous and Aesthetic Surgery,
Northwestern University, Chicago, IL, USA

Series Editor

Jeffrey S. Dover MD FRCPC FRCP
Associate Clinical Professor of Dermatology, Yale University School of Medicine;
Clinical Professor of Surgery, Dartmouth Medical School;
Adjunct Associate Professor of Dermatology, Brown Medical School;
Director, SkinCare Physicians, Chestnut Hill, MA, USA

Associate Editor

Murad Alam MD MSCI
Professor of Dermatology, Otolaryngology, and Surgery;
Chief, Section of Cutaneous and Aesthetic Surgery,
Northwestern University, Chicago, IL, USA

Video Editor

Nazanin Saedi MD
Assistant Professor, Thomas Jefferson University,
Department of Dermatology and Cutaneous Biology,
Philadelphia, PA, USA

ELSEVIER   Edinburgh   London   New York   Oxford   Philadelphia   St Louis   Sydney   Toronto   2016

ELSEVIER

ISBN: 978-0-323-32197-6
ebook ISBN: 978-0-323-34051-9
ebook ISBN: 978-0-323-34052-6

Senior Content Strategist: Belinda Kuhn
Senior Content Development Specialist: Ailsa Laing
Project Manager: Sukanthi Sukumar
Designer: Miles Hitchen
Illustration Manager: Emily Costantino
Multimedia Producer: Jonathan Davis
Marketing Manager: Brian McAllister

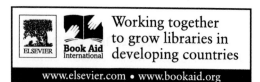

Working together to grow libraries in developing countries

www.elsevier.com • www.bookaid.org

The publisher's policy is to use paper manufactured from sustainable forests

Last digit is the print number: 9 8 7 6 5 4 3 2 1

CONTENTS

Seven years ago we embarked on an effort to produce *Procedures in Cosmetic Dermatology*, a series of high quality, practical, up-to-date, illustrated manuals. Our plan was to provide dermatologists, dermatologic surgeons, and others dedicated to the pursuit of functional knowledge with detailed portable books accompanied by high quality 'how to' DVDs containing all the information they needed to master most, if not all, of the leading edge cosmetic techniques. Thanks to the efforts of world class volume editors, master chapter authors, and the tireless and extraordinary publishing staff at Elsevier, the series has been more successful than any of us could have imagined. Over the past seven years, 15 distinct volumes have been introduced, and have been purchased by thousands of physicians all over the world. Originally published in English, many of the texts have been translated into different languages including Italian, French, Spanish, Chinese, Polish, Korean, Portuguese, and Russian.

Our commitment has always been to ensure that the practical, easy-to-use information conveyed in the series is also extremely up-to-date, incorporating all the latest methods and materials. To that end, given the rapidly changing nature of our subspecialty, the time has now come to inaugurate the third edition. During the next few years, refined, enlarged, and improved texts will be released in a sequential manner. The most time-sensitive books will be revised first, and others will follow.

This series is an ever evolving project. So in addition to third editions of current books, we are introducing entirely new books to cover novel procedures that may not have existed when the series began. Enjoy and keep learning.

Jeffrey S. Dover MD FRCPC FRCP and
Murad Alam MD MSCI

The past couple of decades have seen a revolution in the development of procedures to enhance appearance. A clear trend toward utilizing ever less invasive treatments has been a hallmark of this era in cosmetic dermatology. While many procedures have focused on addressing issues of photoaging that typically affect facial skin, in recent years there has been an emphasis on creating and refining treatments that may impact the appearance of other body sites.

Society currently places a great emphasis on not only youth but also fitness. A well-proportioned and toned physique suggests good health and is felt to be highly desirable, so that diets, exercise regimens, and cosmetic procedures all aimed at creating a more ideal body shape have become extremely popular. However, in the fast paced life of the 21st century, patients demand effective treatments that will provide positive results while necessitating minimal interruption in one's daily life. The challenge to meet those demands has led to a focus within cosmetic dermatology often referred to as non-invasive body sculpting, shaping, or contouring.

We are delighted to share this First Edition of *Body Shaping* with you as part of the 3rd Edition of the *Procedures in Dermatology* series. This text is divided into sections on skin tightening, fat reduction, and cellulite treatments – three of the main goals of non-invasive body contouring. Within each section, you will find a basic science chapter that outlines the etiology of the problem to be addressed and then several chapters detailing the most up-to-date knowledge about various treatment modalities.

This rapidly evolving focus within aesthetic dermatology was initially supported only by anecdotal evidence, but as the field has developed, clinical and translational studies have begun to clarify which procedures work, how well, and why. In every chapter, the authors have provided the most relevant and scientifically grounded evidence possible to provide a clear picture of where we stand in the evolution of these treatments. The text is also supported by outstanding 'how to' videos supplied by the authors, which provide visual instruction and emphasize the clinical pearls provided by our expert authors.

We hope and trust that you will find this volume and the supporting video materials to be instructive, clear, accurate, and thorough.

Jeffrey Orringer MD
Jeffrey S. Dover MD FRCPC FRCP
Murad Alam MD MSCI
April 2015

Murad Alam MD
Professor of Dermatology, Otolaryngology, and Surgery; Chief, Section of Cutaneous and Aesthetic Surgery, Northwestern University, Chicago, IL, USA

Macrene Alexiades-Armenakas, MD PhD
Associate Clinical Professor, Yale University School of Medicine; Director & Founder, Dermatology & Laser Surgery Center of New York, New York, NY, USA

Melissa A. Bogle MD
Director, The Laser and Cosmetic Surgery Center of Houston, Houston, TX; Assistant Clinical Professor, The University of Texas MD Anderson Cancer Center, Houston, TX, USA

Diana Bolotin MD PhD
Assistant Professor, Director of Dermatologic Surgery, Section of Dermatology, University of Chicago, Chicago, IL, USA

Jeffrey S. Dover MD FRCPC FRCP
Associate Clinical Professor of Dermatology, Yale University School of Medicine; Clinical Professor of Surgery, Dartmouth Medical School; Adjunct Associate Professor of Dermatology, Brown Medical School; Director, SkinCare Physicians, Chestnut Hill, MA, USA

Anne Goldsberry MD MBA
Procedural Dermatology Fellow, Laser and Skin Surgery Center of Indiana, Carmel, IN, USA

Heather K. Hamilton
Private Practice, Waldorf Dermatology & Laser Associates, Nanuet, NY, USA

C. William Hanke MD MPH FACP
Director, Micrographic Surgery and Dermatologic Oncology, St. Vincent Hospital, Indianapolis, Indiana; Clinical Professor of Otolaryngology, Indiana University School of Medicine, Indianapolis, Indiana; Visiting Professor of Dermatology, University of Iowa-Carver College of Medicine, Iowa City, Iowa

Camile L. Hexsel MD
Dermatologist and Dermatologic Surgeon, ProHealth Care Medical Associates, Oconomowoc, WI, USA; Investigator of the Brazilian Center for Studies in Dermatology, Porto Alegre, Brazil

Doris Hexsel MD
Dermatologist and Dermatologic Surgeon, Instructor of Cosmetic Dermatology, Department of Dermatology, Pontifícia Universidade Catolica do Rio Grande do Sul (PUC-RS), Porto Alegre, Brazil; Principal Investigator of the Brazilian Center for Studies in Dermatology, Porto Alegre, Brazil

George J. Hruza MD MBA
Medical Director, Laser and Dermatologic Surgery Center; Clinical Professor of Dermatology, Saint Louis University, Saint Louis, MO, USA

Omer Ibrahim MD
Resident, Department of Dermatology, Cleveland Clinic Foundation, Cleveland, OH, USA

Sherrif F. Ibrahim MD PhD
Assistant Professor Dermatology, Division of Dermatologic Surgery, University of Rochester Medical Center, Rochester, NY, USA

James L. Jewell BS
Medical Student; Clinical Research Associate, University of Wollongong, NSW

Mark L. Jewell MD
Associate Clinical Professor Plastic Surgery, Oregon Health Science University, Portland; The Jewell Surgery Center, Eugene, OR, USA

Michael S. Kaminer MD
Associate Clinical Professor of Dermatology, Yale Medical School; Assistant Professor of Dermatology, Brown and Dartmouth Medical Schools; Founding Partner, SkinCare Physicians, Inc., Chestnut Hill, MA, USA

Bruce E. Katz MD
Clinical Professor of Dermatology, The Mount Sinai School of Medicine; Director of the Cosmetic Surgery and Laser Clinic, Mount Sinai Medical Center; Director, Juva Skin and Laser Center, New York, NY, USA

Arielle N. B. Kauvar MD
Director, New York Laser & Skin Care, New York, NY; Clinical Professor of Dermatology, New York University School of Medicine, New York, NY, USA

Emily C. Keller MD
Private Practice, Colorado Springs Dermatology Clinic, Rocky Mountain Laser Center, Colorado Springs, CO, USA

Kathryn M. Kent MD FAAD
Miami Dermatology and Laser Institute, Miami, FL, USA

Misbah Khan, MD FAAD
Assistant Clinical Professor of Dermatology, Weill Cornell Medical Center, New York Presbyterian Hospital; President and Founder M. Khan Dermatology; New York, NY, USA

Nils Krueger PhD
Chief Operating Officer, Rosenpark Research, Darmstadt, Germany

Stefanie Luebberding PhD
Chief Science Officer, Dermatology and Last Surgery Center, New York, NY; now Rosenpark Research, Darmstadt, Germany

Sarah A. Malerich DO
Intern, LewisGale Hospital-Montgomery, Blacksburg, VA, USA

Kira Minkis MD PhD
Department of Dermatology, Northwestern University

Laurel Morton MD
Private Practice, SkinCare Physicians, Chestnut Hill, MA, USA

Jeffrey Orringer MD
Professor and Chief, Division of Cosmetic Dermatology, University of Michigan, Ann Arbor, MI, USA

Rachel N. Pritzker MD
Private Practice, Chicago Cosmetic Surgery and Dermatology, Chicago; Clinical Attending, Cook County Hospital, Chicago, IL, USA

Deanne M. Robinson MD FAAD
Clinical Instructor of Dermatology, Yale Medical School, New Haven, CT; SkinCare Physicians, Chestnut Hill, MA, USA

Anthony M. Rossi MD
Assistant Attending of Dermatology, Memorial Sloan Kettering Cancer Center; Assistant Professor of Dermatology, Weill Cornell Medical College; Assistant Attending, New York Presbyterian Hospital, New York, NY, USA

Adam M. Rotunda MD
Newport Skin Cancer Surgery, Newport Beach, CA; Assistant Clinical Professor of Dermatology, David Geffen School of Medicine (UCLA), Los Angeles, CA; Assistant Clinical Professor of Dermatology, University of California, Irvine, Irvine, CA

Neil S. Sadick MD
Clinical Professor, Department of Dermatology; Weill Medical College of Cornell University, New York, NY; Private Practice, Sadick Dermatology, New York, NY, USA

Nazanin Saedi MD
Assistant Professor, Thomas Jefferson University, Department of Dermatology and Cutaneous Biology, Philadelphia, PA

Roberta Spencer Del Campo
Clinical Lecturer, Division of Cosmetic Dermatology, University of Michigan, Ann Arbor, MI, USA

Robert A. Weiss MD FAAD FACPh
Clinical Associate Professor, Department of Dermatology, University of Maryland; President-Elect, American Society for Laser Medicine and Surgery; Past-President, American Society for Dermatologic Surgery; Director, MD Laser Skin & Vein Institute, Baltimore, MD, USA

To my parents, Mark and Susan Orringer, whose lives are a testament to the beauty, power, and meaning of hard work, kindness, giving back, and always doing the right thing. I could never have hoped for better role models. To my children, Matthew and Katie, for countless moments of pride, inspiration, and laughter – you have both brought me more joy than you will ever know. And especially to my Harvard Medical School classmate, best friend, and wife, Kelly Orringer – your keen mind and inner goodness have always made me view the world in new ways. Thank you for your encouragement, friendship, and love. I love you.

Jeffrey Orringer

To the women in my life: my grandmothers Bertha and Lillian, my mother Nina, my daughters Sophie and Isabel, and especially to my wife Tania – for their never-ending encouragement, patience, support, love and friendship. To my father Mark, a great teacher and role model; to my mentor Kenneth A. Arndt for his generosity, kindness, sense of humor, joie de vivre, and above all else curiosity and enthusiasm.

Jeffrey S. Dover

Elsevier's dedicated editorial staff has made possible the continuing success of this ambitious project. The new team led by Belinda Kuhn have refined the concept while maintaining the series' reputation for quality and cutting-edge relevance. In this, they have been ably supported by the signature high quality illustrations and layouts that are the backbone of each book. We are also deeply grateful to the volume editors, who have generously found time in their schedules, cheerfully accepted our guidelines, and recruited the most knowledgeable chapter authors. And we especially thank the chapter contributors, without whose work there would be no books at all. Finally, I would also like to convey my debt to my teachers, Kenneth Arndt, Jeffrey Dover, Michael Kaminer, Leonard Goldberg, and David Bickers, and my parents, Rahat and Rehana Alam.

Murad Alam

Skin Laxity: Anatomy, Etiology, and Treatment Indications

Omer Ibrahim, Sherrif F. Ibrahim

Key Messages

- Skin laxity is defined as the acquired loose, relaxed state of the skin that develops with age as a result of skin extensibility (stretch) and decreased skin recoil (return to original state after stretch)

- Intrinsic and extrinsic aging cause specific cutaneous changes, such as epidermal thinning, loss of collagen, degradation of elastin, and redistribution of subcutaneous fat, that all lead to significant skin laxity

- Factors that exacerbate skin laxity include advanced age, cumulative ultraviolet light exposure, smoking, menopause, and rapid weight gain

- Non-invasive treatment modalities, such as lasers, radiofrequency and high frequency ultrasound, aim to restore skin elasticity through stimulation of dermal fibroblasts, dermal reorganization, and collagen remodeling. Minimally invasive procedures, such as dermal fillers and autologous fat transfer, aim to restore skin turgor and volume. Surgical procedures such as rhytidectomy and blepharoplasty permanently remove excess or lax skin

Skin laxity is an acquired cutaneous state in which the skin becomes loose and lax secondary to loss of elasticity. Elasticity is defined as the ability of a material to return to its original state after stretching or straining. The amount of strain a material can endure before breakage is referred to as extensibility. Younger skin exhibits resilient elasticity and recoil when under stretch or stress. With age, elasticity begins to decrease at an early time point while extensibility is maintained well into the seventh decade of life, leading to gradual progression of skin slackness.[1]

Anatomy and pathophysiology

The skin is composed of three distinct layers, the epidermis, dermis, and hypodermis or subcutaneous tissue, that all undergo significant alterations as an individual ages (Fig. 1.1), with one manifestation being change in skin elasticity. Cutaneous aging results from the interplay of several intrinsic and extrinsic factors. Intrinsic aging is a naturally occurring process caused by several factors including gradual oxidative damage and reduction in the rate of skin cell replication (resulting in dermal atrophy), elastic fiber degeneration, and loss of hydration, among many other microscopic changes.[1] Extrinsic aging is due to environmental factors such as sun damage and smoking. Chronic ultraviolet (UV) exposure is the major cause of extrinsic aging, otherwise referred to as photoaging. Photoaging, superimposed on intrinsic aging, causes most of the visible age-related changes in the skin.[2]

Pearl 1

As chronic UV exposure is the single most important factor in extrinsic damage to the skin, the importance of mitigation through diligent sunscreen use and other sun-protective behaviors should be stressed to every dermatologic patient.

Epidermis

Although most of the cutaneous alterations that lead to increased skin laxity involve the dermis, changes within all skin layers exacerbate these effects. Alterations in the epidermis render the skin more vulnerable to damaging influences such as UV radiation, desiccation, and external

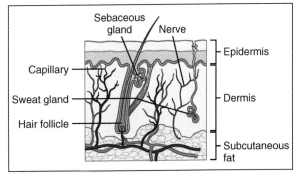

Figure 1.1 Anatomy of the skin

stress, thereby worsening the cumulative effect of the aging process on the underlying structures of the skin. The most striking change in the epidermis is a flattening of the dermal–epidermal junction (DEJ), with effacement of the dermal papillae and rete pegs. This results in less surface area contact between the epidermis and underlying dermis.[2] The decrease in contact surface area between the two skin layers reduces the strength of epidermal attachment to the dermis resulting in an increased tendency to form abrasions and blisters after minor trauma.[3] In addition, the epidermis undergoes a thinning of 10 to 50% between the ages of 30 and 80 years.[4] This atrophy of the epidermis is most notably appreciated in slack eyelid skin, where skin is the thinnest. Furthermore, epidermal stratum corneum lipid concentration declines,[5] leading to a delay in tissue repair and restoration after external stress or trauma.[6] Finally, active epidermal melanocytes are reduced by approximately 10 to 20% per decade, thereby decreasing melanin production and functionally impairing the protective barrier against UV radiation.[2]

Dermis

Specialized junctions connect the dermis and the epidermis and help maintain mechanical integrity and cell-to-cell communication between these two layers. The dermis is the thickest layer of the skin, and is predominantly made up of collagen, elastin, and ground substance composed of glycosaminoglycans and proteoglycans, in addition to cells of the immune system, fibroblasts, blood and lymphatic vessels, nerve fibers, hair follicles and eccrine and apocrine glands. The dermis is further subdivided into two layers. The upper papillary dermal layer contains small, fine, and loose collagen fibrils, while the lower reticular dermis is composed of larger, denser, and interwoven collagen fibrils. The entirety of the dermis provides the skin with its collective tensile strength, elasticity, and malleability.[7]

As cutaneous aging continues, the dermal layer progressively loses volume. The dermis thins by about 20% by late adulthood, and UV exposure tends to exacerbate this thinning.[2] Histologic evaluation of aged skin also shows reduction in cellularity, depletion of vasculature, and loss of elastic fibers and dermal collagen.[8]

Changes in collagen, elastin, and the ground substance cause a loss of flexibility and pliability, and eventual increase in rigidity of the skin. Normally, collagen composes the main structural component of the skin, accounting for 77% of its dry weight.[1] It is stiff, has high tensile strength, and lacks extensibility. With aging, collagen content decreases by approximately 1% per year.[9] Not only does the number of collagen fibrils decrease, but the collagen that remains loses organizational integrity, becomes more compact, and displays increased cross-linking.[2] The increase in cross-linking may be due to a reduction in collagen synthesis, defects in collagen processing, and an increase in collagenases with age.[4]

In addition to collagen, elastic fibers also undergo significant alterations with age. Elastin makes up about 4%

of the skin's dry weight. It is characterized by its elastic extensibility – the ability to stretch under stress but also to recoil and return to its original shape after the stress is removed. Therefore elastin and elastic fibers are inherently important in skin elasticity.[1] It is estimated that as early as young adulthood, elastic fibers diminish in size and number. By late adulthood elastin is degraded, and elastic fibers lose their structural integrity leading to diffuse fragmentation, especially at the DEJ – a condition known as solar elastosis[10] (Fig. 1.2). Furthermore, elastic fibers display more cross-linking, progressive calcification, and at times trans-epidermal extrusion from the dermis (Fig. 1.3). In addition to these structural changes, elastic fibers also endure compositional changes, exhibiting decreases in essential components including elastin and fibrillin.[2] Fibrillin remains abundant in the deeper zones of the dermis; however, it becomes significantly reduced in the upper zone of the dermis.[11] Aged skin displays significant decreases in fibulin-5, an extracellular protein that provides a support base for elastic fibers. Studies have shown

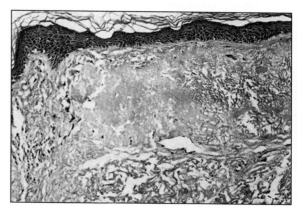

Figure 1.2 Solar elastosis *(from Weedon D, Strutton G, Rubin AI, Weedon D 2010 Weedon's Skin pathology, 3e. Edinburgh, Churchill Livingstone/Elsevier, 2010, p. 341, with permission)*

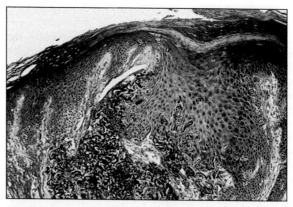

Figure 1.3 Perforating elastosis *(from Disorders of elastic tissue. In Weedon D, Strutton G, Rubin AI, Weedon D 2010 Weedon's skin pathology, 3e. Edinburgh, Churchill Livingstone/Elsevier, p. 341, with permission)*

that a decrease in fibulin-5 expression may be one of the earliest changes, and therefore markers, of cutaneous aging.[12]

Beyond collagen and elastin, the other major structural component of the dermis is the ground substance located between collagen and elastic fibers. It is composed of proteoglycans, glycosaminoglycans (GAGs), and mucopolysaccharides. Of these, hyaluronic acid is most prevalent, and its presence decreases significantly with age – likely due to either decreased hyaluronic acid extractability or decreased hyaluronan secretion. This decrease in hyaluronic acid leads to the formation of altered or less functional ground substance.[2] Overall, as the amount of collagen decreases, the amount of ground substance composed of altered GAGs and proteoglycans increases in photoaged skin.[2] Normally proteoglycans bind about 1000 times their own weight in water and help direct proper collagen deposition, giving youthful skin its tensile strength and supple, voluminous turgor. Therefore, it is no surprise that deleterious age-related changes in the composition of these substances decrease dermal water content, as has been proven on ultrasound imaging, and thereby decrease skin turgor, elasticity and pliability, thus contributing to the appearance of laxity and rhytid formation.[13,14]

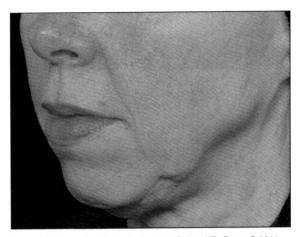

Figure 1.4 Lower facial skin laxity *(from Polder KD, Bruce S 2011 Radiofrequency: thermage. Facial Plast Surg Clin North Am 19(2): 347359, with permission)*

> **Pearl 2**
>
> Skin extensibility can be measured in the clinical setting by lifting and stretching the skin between the thumb and index finger (the pinch test), and skin elasticity can be measured by retraction of the skin (of the eyelid, for example) and observation of the recoil to the original state (the snap test).[1]

Hypodermis

The hypodermis, or subcutaneous tissue, below the dermis is composed mainly of lobules of adipocytes separated by fibrous septa. The hypodermis provides the underlying structures with insulation and cushioning, and comprises the 'scaffolding' that molds the face and body to give them their cosmetic forms.[7]

Among the most striking visual changes to facial skin, is the loss of volume. With age, there is a gradual atrophy and redistribution of the hypodermal fat. The deterioration and redistribution of adipocytes of the subcutaneous layer, in addition to the aforementioned changes in the dermis and epidermis, contributes significantly to the typical appearance and cosmesis of elderly skin[2] (Fig. 1.4). The periorbital area, perioral region, and forehead exhibit reductions in fat content; whereas the jowls, submental area, and nasolabial folds demonstrate prominent increases in fat. Coupled with cumulative gravitational effects over time, this redistribution of fat contributes to sagging and drooping of older skin, causing a shift from the 'inverted triangle'-shaped youthful face to the 'right-side up triangle'-shaped aged face[15] (Fig. 1.5).

The musculature of the face also experiences age-related changes. Muscle cells undergo progressive damage

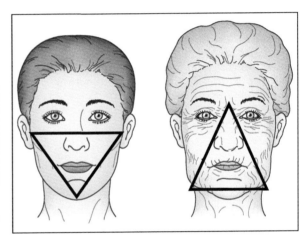

Figure 1.5 Comparison of 'inverted triangle' shape of youthful face and 'right-side up triangle' shape of aged face

and atrophy. The gradual loss in neuromuscular control, along with a reduction in muscle cellularity, exacerbates rhytid formation and saggy skin.[16] Skin laxity and drooping is compounded by changes in the bony structure of the face. All bones in the body, including the facial bones, undergo constant remodeling with a preponderance of resorption later in life, leading to loss of bone mass. The frontal, maxillary, and mandibular bony areas exhibit the majority of bone loss of the face. Facial droopiness is accentuated by the loss of this bony scaffolding and the distinct demarcation between the jaw-line and the neck that is so characteristic and desirable in younger skin, is lost.[17] Table 1.1 summarizes the microscopic alterations seen in each cutaneous layer with advancing age.

Smoking

Smoking aggravates and accelerates the aging process significantly by directly affecting the cells of the dermis and

Table 1.1 Summary of microscopic changes seen in lax skin

Skin layer	Age-induced alterations
Epidermis	Flattening of the dermal–epidermal junction, effacement of the dermal papillae, epidermal thinning, decrease in melanin production
Dermis	Dermal thinning, decrease in cellularity, decrease and loss of organizational integrity of collagen, decrease and degradation of elastin, calcification of elastic fibers, decrease in hyaluronic acid, increase in altered ground substance formation
Hypodermis/ subcutaneous tissue	Atrophy of adipocytes, redistribution of hypodermal fat, loss of muscular cellularity, decrease in neuromuscular control, atrophy of skeletal bone

Pearl 3

The overall appearance of lax skin of the aged face is a reflection of changes in the skin, subcutaneous fat, and bony structure. Therefore, in planning management of these patients, treatment may need to be directed to each of these components separately to achieve maximal results and patient satisfaction.

epidermis, and intensifying the effects of UV radiation on the skin. There is a direct correlation between the number of cigarettes smoked and the severity of skin laxity, wrinkling, and discoloration.[18,19] In general, features of aging are more severe in smokers' skin than among nonsmokers', when controlling for other factors.[20] As in photoaged skin, smoke-damaged skin exhibits elastic fiber fragmentation, but this disarray of elastic fibers penetrates deeper into the dermis.[21] Smoking recruits cutaneous inflammatory cells such as neutrophils with significant elastase activity that cause deep dermal elastosis.[22] Smoking also induces a chronic state of ischemia and oxidative stress that aggravates this elastosis.[18,19] Finally, smoking diminishes water content and estrogen levels in the skin, worsening desiccation, atrophy, and elasticity of aged skin.[18]

Pearl 4

As smoking causes direct cutaneous injury in addition to exacerbating UV-related damage, smoking cessation should be stressed just as strongly as sunscreen use.

Menopause

With life expectancy in the US approaching a norm of 80 years, the average female patient will spend nearly one-third of her life in the post-menopausal state.[23] Therefore, the changes in skin texture and elasticity associated with menopause deserve special attention.

The onset of menopause causes certain alterations in the skin beyond changes associated with chronological aging.[24] Normally, estrogen and progesterone induce proliferation of keratinocytes and collagen synthesis. They inhibit matrix metalloproteinases and induce the production of dermal ground substance.[25] During menopause, estradiol levels decrease by more than 90 percent, accompanied by equally striking decreases in progestin and androgen levels.[26] Decreased dermal collagen levels, decreased skin elasticity, and increased skin extensibility are exacerbated by reduced levels of estrogens. In addition, menopausal skin exhibits significant desiccation and reduced turgor due to decreased sebum levels and reduced water-holding capacity.[2]

Weight gain

The physical strain of rapid weight gain or pregnancy on the skin will cause a brisk expansion and stretching of the skin and underlying tissue. The expanded skin demonstrates higher vascularity, but the dermis and hypodermis are significantly thinned, leading to decreased recoil and tensile strength.[1] Studies have shown that while undergoing expansion, the epidermis maintains its thickness secondary to rapid keratinocyte proliferation; however, the dermis thins during expansion due to slower dermal compensation.[27] Although this extensibility of the skin and ability to lose its recoil are invaluable properties in perioperative tissue expansion for reconstructive purposes, they pose a cosmetic and often a medical problem for individuals left with an accumulation of lax skin after weight loss or pregnancy. In fact, with the recent surge in bariatric surgery, post weight-loss skin reduction surgery has become its own medical subspecialty.

Treatment indications

Although skin laxity is often a purely cosmetic concern to the patient, excess lax skin can pose significant medical consequences in addition to purely aesthetic concerns. For example, dermatochalasis, or redundant eyelid skin, may cause visual field loss, recurrent blepharitis, and entropion with eyelash ptosis resulting in recurrent keratitis.[28] The treatment of skin laxity, whether for medically necessary or aesthetic reasons, has traditionally entailed invasive surgery aimed at removal of excess skin.[29] Over time, newer therapeutic options have evolved to include less invasive light and energy modalities such as lasers, radiofrequency and high frequency ultrasound, that target skin laxity with less trauma and shorter recovery time. Heat-inducing therapies can cause skin tightening through tissue coagulation, liquefaction of adipose tissue, collagen remodeling and stimulation of dermal fibroblasts. These therapies have also been shown to affect reorganization of the reticular dermis and generation of new collagen, leading to increased skin elasticity and skin shrinkage.[30]

Pearl 5

In recent years, patients have been seeking less invasive procedures with shorter recovery periods to address skin laxity. These less invasive heat- or light-based modalities can be combined with minimally invasive surgery to achieve cosmetically desirable results.[30]

References

1. Hussain SH, Limthongkul B, Humphreys TR. The biomechanical properties of the skin. Dermatol Surg 2013;39:2193–203.

2. Yaar M, Gilchrest BA. Aging of skin. In: Wolff K, Goldsmith LA, Katz SI, et al., editors. Fitzpatrick's Dermatology in general medicine. 7th ed. New York: McGraw-Hill; 2008 Online. Available: <http://www.accessmedicine.com>.

3. Kurban RS, Bhawan J. Histologic changes in skin associated with aging. J Dermatol Surg Oncol 1990;16:908.

4. Wulf HC, Sandby-Moller J, Kobayasi T, Gniadecki R. Skin aging and natural photoprotection. Micron 2004;35:185.

5. Elias PM, Ghadially R. The aged epidermal permeability barrier: basis for functional abnormalities. In: Gilchrest BA, editor. Geriatric dermatology. Philadelphia: WB Saunders; 2002. p. 103.

6. Ghadially R, Brown BE, Sequeira-Martin SM, et al. The aged epidermal permeability barrier. Structural, functional, and lipid biochemical abnormalities in humans and a senescent murine model. J Clin Invest 1995;95:2281.

7. Chu DH. Development and structure of skin. In: Wolff K, Goldsmith LA, Katz SI, et al., editors. Fitzpatrick's Dermatology in general medicine. 7th ed. New York: McGraw-Hill; 2008 Online. Available: <http://www.accessmedicine.com>.

8. Gilchrest BA. A review of skin ageing and its medical therapy. Br J Dermatol 1996;135:867.

9. Angel P, Szabowski A, Schorpp-Kistner M. Function and regulation of AP-1 subunits in skin physiology and pathology. Oncogene 2001;20:2413.

10. Rongioletti F. Rebora A Fibroelastolytic patterns of intrinsic skin aging: Pseudoxanthoma-elasticum-like papillary dermal elastolysis and white fibrous papulosis of the neck. Dermatolog 1995;191:19.

11. Halder RM. The role of retinoids in the management of cutaneous conditions in blacks. J Am Acad Dermatol 1998; 39:S98.

12. Kadoya K, Sasaki T, Kostka G, et al. Fibulin-5 deposition in human skin: decrease with ageing and ultraviolet B exposure and increase in solar elastosis. Br J Dermatol 2005;153:607.

13. Scott JE. Proteoglycan-fibrillar collagen interactions. Biochem J 1988;252:313.

14. Gniadecka M, Gniadecka R, Serup J, Sondergaard J. Ultrasound structure and digital image analysis of the subepidermal low echogenic band in aged human skin: diurnal changes and interindividual variability. J Invest Dermatol 1994;102:362.

15. Donofrio LM. Fat distribution: a morphologic study of the aging face. Dermatol Surg 2000;26:1107.

16. Dayan D, Abrahami I, Buchner A, et al. Lipid pigment (lipofuscin) in human perioral muscles with aging. Exp Gerontol 1988;23:97.

17. Ramirez OM, Robertson KM. Comprehensive approach to rejuvenation of the neck. Facial Plast Surg 2001;17:129.

18. Smith JB, Fenske NA. Cutaneous manifestations and consequences of smoking. J Am Acad Dermatol 1996;34:717, quiz 733–734.

19. Joffe I. Cigarette smoking and facial wrinkling. Ann Intern Med 1991;115:659.

20. Davis BE, Koh HK. Faces going up in smoke. A dermatologic opportunity for cancer prevention. Arch Dermatol 1992;128: 1106.

21. Frances C, Boisnic S, Hartmann DJ, et al. Changes in the elastic tissue of the non-sun-exposed skin of cigarette smokers. Br J Dermatol 1991;125:43.

22. Weitz JI, Crowley KA, Landman SL, et al. Increased neutrophil elastase activity in cigarette smokers. Ann Intern Med 1987; 107:680.

23. Mathers CD, Iburg KM, Salomon JA, et al. Global patterns of healthy life expectancy in the year 2002. BMC Public Health 2004;4:66.

24. Wildt L, Sir-Petermann T. Oestrogen and age estimations of perimenopausal women. Lancet 1999;354:224.

25. Verdier-Sevrain S, Bonte F, Gilchrest B. Biology of estrogens in skin: Implications for skin aging. Exp Dermatol 2006;15:83.

26. Nelson JF. The potential role of selected endocrine systems in aging processes. In: Masoro EJ, editor. Handbook of physiology. New York: Oxford University Press; 1995.

27. Johnson TM, Lowe L, Brown MD, et al. Histology and physiology of tissue expansion. J Dermatol Surg Oncol 1993;19(12):1074–8.

28. Cahill KV, Bradley EA, Meyer DR, et al. Functional indications for upper eyelid ptosis and blepharoplasty surgery: a report by the American Academy of Ophthalmology. Ophthalmology 2011;118(12):2510–17.

29. Giampapa VC, Di Bernardo BE. Neck recontouring with suture suspension and liposuction: an alternative for the early rhytidectomy candidate. Aesthetic Plast Surg 1995;19(3): 217–23.

30. Dibernardo BE. The aging neck: a diagnostic approach to surgical and nonsurgical options. J Cosmet Laser Ther 2013; 15(2):56–64.

Lasers and Lights: Skin Tightening

Heather K. Hamilton, Rachel N. Pritzker, Macrene Alexiades-Armenakas

2

Key Messages

- There is increasing demand for nonsurgical approaches to skin tightening on the body without downtime and with minimal risk. Lasers and light-based devices are being developed to meet this demand

- The ideal patient candidate is one with mild to moderate skin laxity and realistic expectations of outcome

- These devices are used extensively and safely on the face. Studies and experienced users have demonstrated their usefulness on the arms, legs, and abdomen

- Similar to other noninvasive devices, continual modifications to treatment protocols improve the clinical outcomes

- Skin-tightening treatments may be easily combined with other noninvasive body contouring devices aimed at fat reduction to achieve optimal results

Introduction

Patient concerns increasingly focus on the clinical signs of aging, including dyspigmentation, redness, wrinkles, and laxity of the skin. Increasingly, patients are dissatisfied with tissue redundancy and textual changes that appear on the abdomen, thighs, and upper arms. Traditionally, treatment for such concerns required surgical intervention and involved abdominoplasty, brachioplasty, and liposuction. More recently, technological advances have evolved in the direction of noninvasive body contouring and skin tightening. Although outcomes may not be as dramatic as surgical intervention, the favorable side effect profile and minimal downtime associated with noninvasive procedures have generated high demand from patients. Research and development within this realm has predominantly focused on facial and neck skin tightening, with less emphasis off the face.

Radiofrequency, ultrasound, lasers, and broadband light sources are among the devices most widely used. Clinical improvement of facial rhytides was initially noted when treating other aspects of photoaging with lasers. This finding led to histologic and clinical confirmation of neocollagenesis and rhytid reduction following treatment with lasers in the visible, near-infrared, and mid-infrared spectrum.[1-5] Among the early lasers and light sources, the KTP laser (532 nm), PDL (585 nm and 595 nm), IPL (515–1200 nm), Nd:YAG (1064 nm Q-switched, 1064 nm long-pulsed, 1319 nm, and 1320 nm), diode (980 nm and 1450 nm), and Er:glass (1540 nm) were all found to have some efficacy for facial nonablative resurfacing. However, mid-infrared devices, due to the deeper penetration of their longer wavelengths and lesser absorption by epidermal melanin, were generally found to be the most effective for deeper rhytides and acne scarring after a series of treatments.[5,6] Near-infrared broadband devices have yielded significant reduction of rhytides and skin laxity of the face and neck, with a histologic correlation of both neocollagenesis and neoelastogenesis.[7,8]

Research using lasers and light-based technologies for rhytid reduction or laxity reduction on the body are limited. One important challenge for the investigator is differentiating between skin laxity and cellulite. The focus in this chapter is on the treatment of rhytides and skin laxity, termed 'skin tightening', on the body using lasers and light-based technologies.

Proposed mechanism of action

'Skin laxity' describes loose or redundant skin, with the appearance of prominent skin folds. On the body the most commonly affected areas are the upper arms, thighs, and abdomen. These visible changes are a result of the multifactorial process of skin aging, including both extrinsic and intrinsic factors. Intrinsic factors within the human dermis include loss of collagen, degeneration of the elastic fiber network, and loss of hydration. Extrinsic factors include ultraviolet exposure and the accumulation of elastotic material within the dermis (solar elastosis).[9] Further, skin laxity resulting from mechanical stretching of skin from pregnancy or extreme weight, muscle, or body mass fluctuations may be cosmetically distressing. The goal of noninvasive tissue tightening is to reverse these changes by rebuilding the collagen and elastic scaffold of the dermis.

The mechanism of action of all noninvasive energy devices aimed at skin tightening is deep heating of the tissue. It has been documented that when collagen is heated to 65–70 °C irreversible denaturation of the triple helix occurs with subsequent recoil and contraction.[10,11] It is then hypothesized that the long-term skin-tightening effects are a consequence of this thermal damage initiating long-term remodeling of the dermis, with new collagen deposition and fibroplasia.[12–15] The way in which collagen is heated differs for each category of noninvasive skin-tightening device.

Pearl 1

The infrared light-emitting devices target water as a chromophore and subsequently heat the surrounding collagen to elicit neocollagenesis and, in some cases, neoelastogenesis, associated with clinical improvement in rhytides and skin laxity.

Among laser and light devices, those in the infrared wavelength spectrum have been found to be the most effective in obtaining any degree of skin tightening. Devices in the mid-infrared spectrum are weakly absorbed by water within the dermis. Infrared devices within the wavelengths of 1000–1800 nm are able to penetrate deeper into the dermis than lasers in the visible light spectrum due to their longer wavelength and decreased absorption by melanin and hemoglobin (Fig. 2.1). Longer

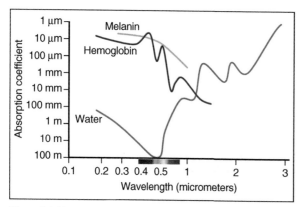

Figure 2.1 Absorption of light by discrete chromophores in tissue (adapted from Willey A, Lee KK. Broadband light and laser. In: Alam M, Dover J, editors. Non-surgical skin tightening and lifting. Elsevier; 2009, with permission)

Pearl 2

The use of epidermal cooling is essential to prevent bulk heating and injury to the epidermis.

---

wavelengths in the infrared spectrum, such as 2940 nm Er:YAG and 10,600 nm CO_2 lasers, are strongly absorbed by water which significantly limits their depth of penetration. Gentle volumetric heating of collagen from the energy absorbed by water may be achieved when laser/light is administered over longer pulse durations. Mechanisms to cool the epidermis are necessary when treating the dermis with infrared devices to prevent bulk heating related damage to the skin's surface.

Infrared devices

Clinical studies of infrared devices demonstrate immediate and delayed collagen changes post-procedure. Dermal collagen denaturation was seen on transmission electron microscopy from abdominoplasty skin samples immediately after irradiation with an infrared device (Titan, Cutera Inc., Brisbane, CA). Higher fluences correlated with deeper tissue injury, and the depth of maximal damage occurred at 1–2 mm.[16] Although not fully understood, this immediate injury leads to subsequent wound remodeling over time, which is believed to create the skin-tightening effect that peaks over a 3–6-month period. In human skin treated using a 1450 nm flashlamp-excited Er: glass laser, biopsies obtained 2 months post-irradiation showed zones of dermal fibroplasia with increased numbers of fibroblasts observed at the depths corresponding to the initial thermal-induced changes.[13] In an animal study, skin treated with an infrared laser device showed a significant increase in both type I and type III collagen at 45 days after irradiation. The type I collagen density remained significantly increased on histological examination 90 days after treatment, suggesting neocollagenesis.[15] Furthermore, these investigators found similar findings in human skin. In both sun-protected and sun-exposed skin, there was a significant increase relative to controls in type III collagen and elastin persisting at the last data point taken 90 days post-procedure.[15]

Four devices that are versions of the Titan system have been marketed to promote skin tightening on the body (Table 2.1). The Titan device (Cutera Inc., Brisbane, CA)

Table 2.1 Devices using broadband infrared (IR) light source for skin tightening on the body

Device/manufacturer	Wavelengths	Handpiece size	Cooling
StarLux-IR, Lux-IR (Palomar)	850–1350 nm	12 × 28 mm	Sapphire contact cooling
Titan (Cutera)	1100–1800 nm	15 × 10 mm and 30 × 10 mm	Sapphire contact cooling
SkinTyte (Sciton)	800–1400 nm	1.5 × 4.5 cm	Sapphire contact cooling
VelaShape (Syneron)	700–2000 nm	30 × 30 mm and 40 × 40 mm	None

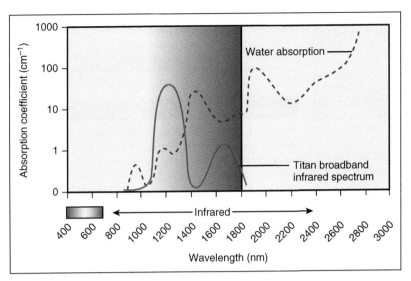

Figure 2.2 The tailored spectrum delivered by the infrared broadband light device (Titan). Wavelengths of 1100–1800 nm provide a penetration depth of up to 2 mm, since the most strongly absorbed wavelengths in the range of 1400–1800 nm are attenuated *(from Tazi E, Alster TS. Noninvasive tissue tightening. In: Kaminer MS, Arndt KA, Dover JS, et al, editors. Atlas of Cosmetic Surgery, 2nd ed. Philadelphia: Elsevier; 2009, with permission)*

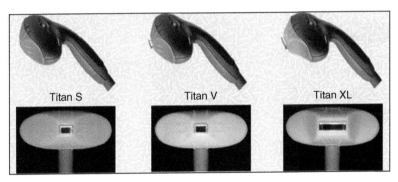

Figure 2.3 Examples of the handpiece and their respective diameters for treatment of various size areas with the infrared broadband device *(Titan; courtesy of Cutera Inc.)*

is an infrared light device emitting the spectrum from 1100 to 1800 nm. These wavelengths have a moderate level of water absorption and therefore can safely heat the dermis over a longer pulse duration when coupled with epidermal cooling mechanisms (Fig. 2.2). The Titan XL (3 cm^2 spot size) has a maximum fluence of 50 J/cm^2 while the Titan S and V (1.5 cm^2 spot size) have a maximum fluence of 65 J/cm^2 (Fig. 2.3). The pulse duration ranges up to 8.1 seconds. The handpiece is equipped with a sapphire window for pre-, parallel-, and post-cooling.[17] A mobile technique has been developed which allows the use of 30% higher fluences, painlessly and safely, while maintaining efficacy in laxity improvement on the face and neck.[8,18] The Titan is the only nonablative device shown to induce neocollagenesis and neoelastogenesis, which may explain its efficacy in treating both rhytides and laxity.[15]

The second infrared lamp device (Lux-IR Fractional, Palomar Medical Inc., Burlington, MA) uses a near-infrared halogen lamp with a filtered spectrum of 850 to 1350 nm but with a unique fractionated handpiece. The handpiece with a spot size of 12 × 28 mm includes a skin surface cooling sapphire tip and a patterned optical window. The window contains an array of 21 apertures, each with a diameter of 3 mm, which facilitates delivery

of the infrared energy within multiple spatially confined thermal lesions within the dermis. The device can deliver a total fluence of up to 200 J/cm^2 over a possible 10-second pulse duration.[19]

Thirdly, the SkinTyte II filter may be inserted onto Sciton's broadband light (BBL) device (Sciton, Palo Alto, CA) to emit a broadband infrared spectrum of 800–1400 nm. Fluence ranges from 0 to 60 J/cm^2 for the stationary technique and power ranges from 0 to 25 W/cm^2 for the mobile technique. (These techniques are elaborated further in a later section.) Cutoff filters of 590, 695 or 800 nm may be employed with the mobile delivery method. Typical starting fluence for the stationary method is 40 J/cm^2. Starting power setting for the mobile delivery is recommended at approximately 10 W/cm^2. There is a sapphire tip to provide contact cooling.

Infrared light and diode lasers have been combined with bipolar radiofrequency to synergistically heat and therefore tighten the skin. This device, called the Vela-Shape® (Syneron, Medical Ltd, Israel), has demonstrated tightening on both the arm and post-partum abdominal skin utilizing a combination of bipolar radiofrequency, infrared light, vacuum, and massage. The combination of light and radiofrequency is termed electro-optical synergy (ELOS) technology. The radiofrequency uses emission between 3 kHz and 1 MHz which generates heat by movement of electrons abiding by the principle of Ohm's law. The use of the infrared light is able to first superficially heat the dermis as described previously, thereby lowering the impedance of the target tissue and allowing for potentially enhanced efficacy of the radiofrequency current. The vacuum device folds the epidermis and dermis between the two electrodes, allowing for less total energy to be employed and decreasing the risk of epidermal damage over unfolded skin.[11,20]

A near-infrared device (NIR, Harmony, Alma Lasers) is in clinical trials (Alexiades-Armenakas, personal communication) for treatment of skin laxity of the thighs and abdomen. This near-infrared broadband light device has an output of 800–1600 nm, power output of 1–100 W, and a spot size of 18 cm². Epidermal cooling is provided by a sapphire tip. Typical settings include 50 W for the delivery of approximately 30 kJ per 100 cm² treatment area using a mobile technique (Alexiades-Armenakas, personal communication).

Patient selection

The ideal candidate for noninvasive tightening procedures has mild to moderate laxity and has excluded surgical tightening procedures at the present time.

Pearl 3

Patient selection is essential with these noninvasive devices. Expected results versus surgical outcomes should be reviewed and expectations managed prior to instituting treatment.

It is critical to discuss with patients that the degree of cosmetic enhancement with noninvasive procedures is typically modest at best and that some patients do not obtain appreciable improvement. Management of expectations is paramount for patient satisfaction, and it should be clarified that these devices are reserved for those patients who have ruled out plastic surgery. Pregnancy is a contraindication. Special attention should be paid to patients with implants or prior surgeries in the treatment area, an indwelling pacemaker or defibrillator, a history of keloids, diabetes, or vitiligo, those on a photosensitizing drug, or taking isotretinoin within the past 6 months. Treatments should not be performed if any rash is seen in the treatment area. Infrared devices are generally safe for darker pigmented skin types or tanned skin, though a test spot is generally recommended. It is of the utmost importance to take detailed pre-procedure standardized photographs.

Pearl 4

Infrared devices are generally safe for darker pigmented skin types or tanned skin, though a test spot is always recommended.

Pearl 5

Standardized pre- and post-procedure photographs are strongly encouraged to track efficacy.

Treatment course

After a full discussion about the risks, benefits, side effects, and alternative treatments, and the opportunity for the patient to ask questions, a signed written informed consent should be obtained. The treatment area is then cleaned. Pre-procedure standardized photographs should be taken. These photos may be valuable in showing the patient improvement at follow-up visits, particularly because results may be subtle. It is important that the photographic technique and lighting are consistent in 'before' and 'after' photographs. Any hair at the treatment site should be removed to allow for complete contact with the handpiece. The use of anesthetics is not recommended, as patient feedback is important for safety.

Titan

The Titan device (Cutera Inc., Brisbane, CA) provides dermal heating at a depth of 1–2 mm. It emits noncoherent, broadband infrared light at 1100–1800 nm with a filter for the strongly water absorbing wavelengths of 1400–1500 nm. There are two spot sizes to choose from depending on the size of the treatment area: 1.5 × 1 cm and 3 × 1 cm. The fluence ranges from 5 to 50 J/cm² for the 3 cm spot size and up to 65 J/cm² for the 1.5 cm spot size. A fluence of 36–46 J/cm² is recommended for treatments on the body. Using the stationary technique, the recommended starting fluence is 36 J/cm², and 45–46 J/cm² with the mobile technique.[8] The patient should experience a heat sensation, but not burning. The fluence should be reduced if the patient reports extreme heat, discomfort, or a burning sensation. Great care should be taken to apply adequate aqueous gel so that full contact of the sapphire tip is maintained with the gel and skin surface. Special care to maintain contact should be taken at bony prominences. The treatment parameters are adjusted until immediate erythema and mild edema in the treatment area is seen without evidence of epidermal disruption (with blister formation) (Fig. 2.4). The pulse duration is automatically adjusted based on the selected fluence and is displayed on the screen. There is pre-, parallel-, and post-cooling provided by a temperature-regulated sapphire crystal window.

The patient, operator, and everyone in the room must wear appropriate protective goggles. A layer of ultrasound gel is applied to the treatment area, approximately 3 mm thick. Refrigerating the gel prior to use increases patient comfort. Adequate pressure must be applied to ensure full contact of the handpiece with the skin during the entire pulse. Using the stationary technique, the handpiece is then moved the width of the window for the subsequent

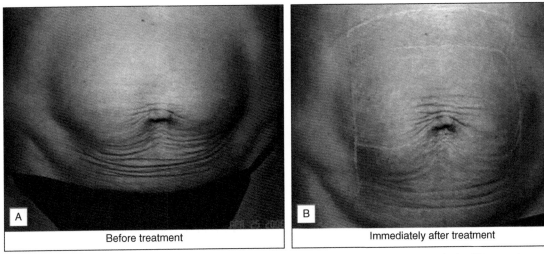

A	B
Before treatment	Immediately after treatment

Figure 2.4 Expected erythema and mild edema seen immediately after treatment with a broadband infrared device *(Titan; courtesy of Cutera Inc.)*

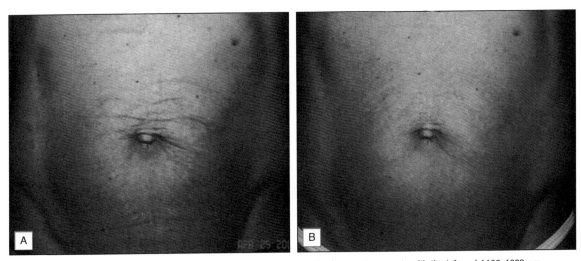

Figure 2.5 Abdominal skin tightening. **(A)** At baseline and **(B)** at 6 months following two treatments with the infrared 1100–1800 nm broadband device (Titan) at 42–43 J/cm², 467 total pulses *(courtesy of Jacqueline Calkin)*

pulse. Typical treatment protocols include 3 to 4 passes of adjacent exposures. The number of pulses varies depending the surface area, but on the abdomen may be estimated at around 300–450.[21] Using the mobile technique, each pulse is administered in an oval or circular motion extending approximately one handpiece width laterally and vertically. The pulses are delivered in linear succession in groups of 4–5 pulses with 6–8 passes per pulse group before moving to a new area.[8] Two to four treatments are commonly performed at 1–3-month intervals.[8,22] The endpoint is visible erythema, mild edema, and skin firmness, and passes are completed until this is achieved (see Fig. 2.4). If the patient reports an intolerable level of discomfort, the operator should release the foot switch, which will end the exposure but keep the handpiece in contact with skin until the discomfort resolves by utilizing the contact cooling. Then, the fluence may be reduced and/or the handpiece moved to the next treatment spot. There should be no overlap of the pulses to minimize the risk of excessive bulk heating. Clinical results are typically appreciated from 2 weeks following the first treatment, with the final outcome appreciable at 6 months following the last treatment (Fig. 2.5).

Lux-IR

The Lux-IR (Lux-IR Fractional™, Cynosure, Westford, MA) emits light from 850 nm to 1350 nm via a fractionated window that contains an array of 21 apertures, each with a diameter of 3 mm. The handpiece has a spot size of 12 × 28 mm and a sapphire contact cooling tip. A contact sensor allows pulse delivery only when the skin is in full contact with the cooling tip. For treatment on the abdomen and thighs, settings may be as follows: 2–3 seconds of pre-cooling, 3.5 second pulse duration, fluences of 40–80 J/cm^2, and 2 seconds post-cooling.[19]

The patient, operator, and anyone else in the room must wear appropriate protective goggles. To aid with comfort, the SheerCool Roller™ may be rolled over the treatment area for 10–15 seconds prior to treatment. Good contact of the handpiece with the skin during the entire pulse is paramount. At the end of each pulse, the handpiece should be moved to the adjacent skin without overlap. Treatments typically include 1–4 passes with at least 2 minutes between passes. When treating the arms, the entire circumference of the upper arm should be treated.[19] If the patient feels any pain or a burning sensation, the foot pedal should be released to interrupt the pulse, but the treatment window should remain in contact with the skin to take advantage of the contact cooling.[19]

SkinTyte II

SkinTyte (Sciton, Palo Alto, CA) emits a broadband infrared spectrum of 800–1400 nm. The spot size is 15 × 45 mm and there are adapters to treat smaller areas. Fluence ranges from 0 to 60 J/cm^2 for the stationary technique and power ranges from 0 to 25 W/cm^2 for the mobile technique. Cutoff filters of 590, 695 or 800 nm may be employed with the mobile delivery method. Typical starting fluence for the stationary method is 40 J/cm^2. Starting power setting for the mobile delivery is recommended at approximately 10 W/cm^2. There is a sapphire tip to provide contact cooling.

A thin layer of gel at room temperature is applied to the treatment area. A SkinTyte II filter is inserted into the BBL handpiece and the Smooth Adapter is attached to cover the edges of the crystal. Operators may use a stationary approach or a mobile technique. The mobile technique was developed to make the treatment more tolerable, reduce treatment time, and maximize energy delivery without compromising efficacy. This approach was developed by one of the authors with prior radio-frequency and infrared technologies.[23] It involves moving the handpiece slowly in a circular motion. For the stationary technique, a fluence output of 40 J/cm^2 is recommended with an 800-nm cutoff filter. For the mobile technique, a starting power output of 10 W/cm^2 is recommended with any of three filters including 590, 695 or 800 nm. The endpoint is a surface temperature of 40–42 °C. Sciton recommends three to six treatments performed at 2- to 4-week intervals.

VelaShape

The ELOS device VelaShape (Syneron Medical Ltd, Israel) employs infrared (IR), bipolar radiofrequency (RF), vacuum, and mechanical massage. It has FDA clear-

ance for temporary reduction in the appearance of cellulite and for temporary circumferential reduction but has also been found to produce skin tightening. There are two applicators, the VSmooth and the VContour. The VSmooth has a spot size of 40 × 40 mm, an RF power of up to 60 W, and an IR power of up to 35 W. The VContour has a spot size of 30 × 30 mm, an RF power of up to 23 W, and an IR power of up to 20 W. They both emit broadband IR light of 700–2000 nm and have a vacuum with pulsed 180–380 mbar. Mechanical massage is only part of the VSmooth. The VSmooth is recommended for treatments on the thighs, buttocks, and abdomen while the VContour is recommended for the arms, calf, bra-line, and flanks. Recommended parameters for both applicators are the following for cellulite improvement and circumference reduction, respectively: IR 2–3, RF 3, and vacuum 1–2; and IR 1, RF 3, and vacuum 2–3. It is recommended to reduce the IR level for deep treatment, for dark or tanned skin, or when stacking pulses. It is suggested to set the RF to the highest level tolerated. The vacuum should be gradually increased in subsequent sessions, increased for deep treatment, and reduced on sensitive areas or loose skin. If the patient complains of pain, it is recommended that the vacuum is reduced. If stinging occurs the operator should reduce the RF, and if the patient complains of excessive heat, reduce the IR.

Immediately prior to the procedure, a thin layer of treatment lotion is applied to the treatment area. Each area is divided into strips as wide as the applicator for repeated passes until the external temperature reaches 40–42 °C. If the area is large, it should be divided into two sections, as it is easier to reach and maintain the endpoint temperature desired for the skin-tightening effect. Regardless of device, maintenance at 42 °C is typically required for a minimum of 5 minutes for clinical improvement to be attained. Maintaining full contact with the skin throughout the entire pulse is important. It is recommended to work in motion to achieve the best contact – backward and forward motions for the VSmooth applicator and stacks for the VContour applicator. The treatment area is then left to cool until it reaches about 37 °C at which point it is treated again to a skin surface endpoint of 40–42 °C. A handheld laser thermometer monitors surface temperature. Typically, four to six treatments are performed at weekly intervals. For maintenance, monthly treatments that may gradually be stretched out to one every 3–6 months are recommended.

Near infrared

Recently, a near-infrared device (NIR, Harmony, Alma Lasers) has been in clinical trials for the treatment of skin laxity of the thighs and abdomen (Alexiades-Armenakas, personal communication; see Fig. 2.6). This near-infrared broadband light device emits wavelengths of 800–1600 nm, with a power output of 50–100 W, and a spot size of 18 cm^2. Epidermal cooling is provided by the temperature-regulated sapphire tip. A thin layer of

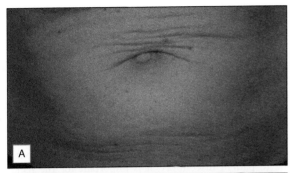

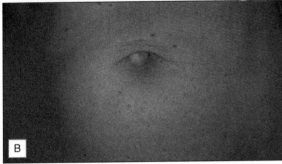

Figure 2.6 Treatment of abdominal skin rhytides and laxity with a novel near-infrared (800–1600 nm) broadband light device (NIR, Alma Lasers) **(A)** at baseline and **(B)** at 1 month following three monthly sessions at 50 W and total energy delivery of 30 kJ *(courtesy of Macrene Alexiades-Armenakas)*

aqueous gel is applied to the skin. Typical parameters are a power level of 50 W with a mobile delivery method.[8] The handpiece is moved in an oval motion approximately one handpiece-width laterally, superiorly and inferiorly over an approximately 10 cm^2 area until confluent mild erythema is attained. The patient should report feeling warmth or heat, but not a burning sensation. The patient should be instructed to report whether a burning sensation is felt. Once the desired clinical endpoint of confluent erythema is achieved, the aforementioned procedure should be repeated in the adjacent 10 cm^2 region of skin. The process is repeated for an entire anatomic region (e.g. abdomen) until delivery of 30 kJ is achieved per 100 cm^2 treatment area (Alexiades-Armenakas, manuscript in preparation). The handpiece is then applied in the mobile fashion throughout the treatment zone and moved from area to area in order to maintain confluent erythema, and should be continually moved if the patient reports extreme heat, discomfort or burning sensations, until 30 kJ is delivered. Great care should be taken to apply adequate aqueous gel so that full contact of the sapphire tip is maintained with the gel and skin surface. A clinical result is noted at the earliest 2 weeks following the first treatment and the patient may experience additional improvements until the final outcome is noted approximately 6 months following the final treatment. Typically, two to four monthly treatments.

Expected outcomes

Data is limited for noninvasive light and laser devices for skin tightening on the body. In a multicenter clinical perspectives report describing use of the Titan device on facial and nonfacial sites, one patient's abdomen was treated twice with marked (51–75%) improvement at 1.5 months' follow-up and one patient's arms were treated twice with marked improvement at 3 months' follow-up.[22] In a study of 20 female patients with mild to very loose aged upper arm skin, minimal improvement was found after two treatments with the Titan device. A statistically significant decrease in arm circumference of 0.38 cm was achieved but blinded assessors of before and after photos did not observe a statistically significant improvement in appearance.[24] In a study of 303 patients, 25 patients were treated on two occasions 2 months apart on their abdomen, legs, or buttocks. Each treatment consisted of four passes using a fluence of 44–48 J/cm^2 for the abdomen, 42–46 J/cm^2 for the medial thighs, and 44–50 J/cm^2 for the buttocks. The endpoint was patient satisfaction. Forty percent of patients rated their degree of satisfaction as 'very satisfactory', 20% as 'satisfactory', and 40% as 'unsatisfactory'. The degree of satisfaction was lower than the level of satisfaction reported by patients who had had treatments on their face or neck. No objective measures were used to assess results in this study.[25]

In a study of the VelaShape, 20 women who had had at least one pregnancy and were at least 9 months postpartum with resultant sagging skin, cellulite, and skin irregularities or modified contours in their abdomen were treated weekly for 5 weeks. Twelve of the participants elected to also have their buttocks treated, and the other eight elected to have their thighs treated. Statistically significant reductions in circumference and cellulite were reported. The distribution of the subjective and objective assessments of the skin's texture and tightness at the follow-up visit is portrayed figuratively. Physician assessment found 29% of the treatment areas showed good improvement, 58% showed moderate improvement, and 13% showed slight improvement. Eight percent of patients graded their improvement as excellent, 26% rated their improvement as good, 32% as moderate, 29% as slight, and 5% as none.[26] In another study of the VelaShape, 19 subjects underwent five weekly treatments to the upper arms and 10 subjects underwent four weekly treatments to the abdomen and flanks. The majority of treatments were performed at level 3 RF, level 2 IR, and level 1–2 vacuum. The investigators found a statistically significant reduction in the circumference of treatment areas. They reported that 47.3% of patients whose arms were treated were either slightly satisfied, satisfied, or very satisfied at 1 month follow-up and 80% of patients who underwent treatments to their abdomen were either satisfied, very satisfied, or extremely satisfied at 1 month follow-up. Skin-tightening results were not specifically reported.[20] Overall, the improvement in contour including cellulite and circumference reduction are likely due, at least in part, to a skin-tightening effect as the purported mechanism of action of this combination technology is the heating and subsequent remodeling of the collagen within the dermis.

Safety

The incidence of side effects and complications with the infrared devices for skin-tightening treatment is low. In general, to avoid complications with these types of devices, the operator must be aware of the amount of heat being transferred and ways to avoid excessive heating. Immediately post-procedure, there is mild erythema and edema seen within the entire treated area (see Fig. 2.4). This is short lived, usually fading within a few hours, but has on occasion lasted a few days without complication.[22]

Pearl 6

The expected endpoint is confluent mild erythema and mild edema of the treated area.

Since the goal of the procedure is sustained dermal heating, post-procedure cooling is not necessary unless an area is overly erythematous or painful to the patient.

Pearl 7

Continual monitoring of the tissue response is vital for safety. Employing a mobile technique has greatly improved safety and minimized the risk of thermal injury.[8]

Pearl 8

If the patient reports pain or intense heat, the operator must stop the emission of energy and allow the cooling device to remain on the surface of the skin.

The most common adverse event due to overheating is a superficial burn. In a study of 25 patients undergoing facial skin tightening with the broadband infrared device (Titan, Brisbane, CA), three patients had small, superficial second-degree burns. With the appropriate aftercare, these healed without sequale.[17] A mobile pulse application where circular movements are performed for each pulse was employed in one case series to the face and neck, and there were no adverse events noted. This suggests a possible adjustment to treatment protocols in order to avoid vesiculation and blistering.[8] Full thickness permanent scars have been documented with an infrared device. Scars included single hyperpigmented rectangular flat areas, multiple hyperpigmented and hypopigmented elevated rectangular areas, and multiple extensive atrophic and hypertrophic rectangular areas with both hyperpigmentation and hypopigmentation. These scars were most prominent over bony surfaces.[27] Possible mechanisms contributing to these burns include improper handpiece positioning, errors in omitting the use of gel, excessive treatment parameters, and increased heat over bony structures with consequent nonselective heating of the tissue. Ways to minimize the risk of complications include ensuring proper cooling, having a checklist to ensure proper placement of the gel and treatment settings, using caution over bony prominences, avoiding pulse stacking, and aborting the energy delivered if the patient gives feedback of excessive heat. If a user stops the energy within a pulse due to patient discomfort, it is important for the handpiece to remain on the skin so that the sapphire tip handpiece may continue to sufficiently cool the area in question.

Multi-modality procedures

Noninvasive skin-tightening devices, including the infrared tightening devices discussed in this chapter, may be used as an adjunct to liposuction or other fat reduction procedures. Post-operative skin laxity is a not an uncommon complaint following liposuction, which led to the use by some clinicians of simultaneous laser-assisted tightening during liposuction. Although studies are lacking, noninvasive skin-tightening devices would theoretically be of benefit for improving skin laxity that may result from surgical fat reduction.

CASE STUDY 1

Patient JY is a 43-year old white female who presents complaining of loose, creased skin on her abdomen. She first noticed the condition after her two pregnancies, but it has worsened over time. She reports being embarrassed when she is sitting or leaning forward, as this accentuates numerous wrinkled skin folds. As JY is extremely thin and exercises regularly, she has a very low BMI, which rules out liposuction and makes abdominoplasty less apt to yield a successful outcome. The patient is not willing to pursue surgery, and instead is interested in nonsurgical options to improve the appearance of her abdominal rhytides and laxity.

Physical examination is significant for extensive crepe-like rhytides and moderate laxity of the abdomen extending from the periumbilical region to the suprapubic region.

Education is provided to patient JY on the various treatment options, including no treatment, surgical options, and laser and light-based treatments. Given the lack of observable fat, she is not a candidate for liposuction. Following consultation and discussion of the treatment options, the patient proceeds with treatment with a broadband infrared device. She undergoes three treatments at monthly intervals. The parameters are as follows: near-infrared (800–1600 nm, 50 W, 18 cm^2 spot size; NIR, Alma Lasers). Each treatment was painless with minimal erythema and no adverse events.

Patient JY achieved significant improvement in the degree of creasing and skin laxity of her mid-to-lower abdomen. She tolerated it well with no complications (see Fig. 2.6).

CASE STUDY 2

Patient LB is a 49-year old white female who presents complaining of irregularities of the contours of her abdomen. She has been treated with cryolipolysis in the past and would now like a smoother appearance to the surface texture. She reports that the irregularity of her abdominal texture has so concerned her that she has avoided wearing a two-piece bathing suit. LB is very thin and exercises regularly. She is not interested in plastic surgery, and instead is only interested in nonsurgical options to improve the appearance of her abdominal skin.

Physical examination is significant for textural irregularities of the surface of the mid-abdomen and moderate skin laxity. Minimal subcutaneous fat is appreciable.

A discussion with LB of the various treatment options, including no treatment, surgical options, liposuction, and laser and light-based treatments, is conducted. Given the minimal fat present, liposuction and laser-assisted liposuction are discussed; however, the patient prefers a noninvasive form of treatment. Following consultation and discussion of the treatment options, the patient proceeds with treatment with infrared broadband light. She undergoes three treatments at monthly intervals. The parameters are as follows: near-infrared (800–1100 nm, 46 J/cm^2, mobile technique; Titan, Cutera Lasers). Each treatment was painless with minimal erythema and no adverse events.

Patient LB achieves significant improvement in the contour irregularities and skin laxity of her mid-to-lower abdomen. She tolerated her treatment series well with no complications.

References

1. Goldberg D, Tan M, Dale Sarradet M, Gordon M. Nonablative dermal remodeling with a 585-nm, 350-microsec, flashlamp pulsed dye laser: clinical and ultrastructural analysis. Dermatol Surg 2003;29:161–3.
2. Goldberg DJ. New collagen formation after dermal remodeling with an intense pulsed light source. J Cutan Laser Ther 2000; 2:59–61.
3. Fatemi A, Weiss MA, Weiss RA. Short-term histologic effects of nonablative resurfacing: results with a dynamically cooled millisecond-domain 1320 nm Nd:YAG laser. Dermatol Surg 2002;28(2):172–6.
4. Dayan SH, Vartanian AJ, Menaker G, et al. Nonablative laser resurfacing using the long-pulse (1064-nm) Nd:YAG laser. Arch Facial Plast Surg 2003;5:310–15.
5. Alexiades-Armenakas MR, Dover JS, Arndt KA. The spectrum of laser skin resurfacing: nonablative, fractional, and ablative laser resurfacing. J Am Acad Dermatol 2008;58:719–37.
6. Alam M, Dover JS, Arndt K. Energy delivery devices for cutaneous remodeling lasers, lights, and radio waves. Arch Dermatol 2003;139(10):1351–60.
7. Kameyama K. Histological and clinical studies on the effects of low to medium level infrared light therapy on human and mouse skin. J Drugs Dermatol 2008;7(3):230–4.
8. Alexiades-Armenakas M. Assessment of the mobile delivery of infrared light (1100–1800 nm) for the treatment of facial and neck skin laxity. J Drugs Dermatol 2009;8(3):221–6.
9. Uitto J. The role of elastin and collagen in cutaneous aging: intrinsic aging versus photoexposure. J Drugs Dermatol 2008; 7(2 Suppl.):s12–16.
10. Arnoczky SP, Aksan A. Thermal modification of connective tissues: basic science considerations and clinical applications. J Am Acad Orthop Surg 2000;8:305–13.
11. Alster TS, Lupton JR. Nonablative cutaneous remodeling using radiofrequency devices. Clin Dermatol 2007;25:487–91.
12. Orringer JS, Voorhees JJ, Hamilton T, et al. Dermal matrix remodeling after nonablative laser therapy. J Am Acad Dermatol 2005;53(5):775–82.
13. Ross EV, Sajben FP, Hsia J, et al. Nonablative skin remodeling: selective dermal heating with a mid-infrared laser and contact cooling combination. Lasers Surg Med 2000;26(2):186–95.
14. Tanaka Y, Matsuo K, Yuzuriha S, Shinohara H. Differential long-term stimulation of type I versus type III collagen after infrared irradiation. Dermatol Surg 2009;35(7): 1099–104.
15. Tanaka Y, Matsuo K, Yuzuriha S. Long-term evaluation of collagen and elastin following infrared (1100 to 1800 nm) irradiation. J Drugs Dermatol 2009;8(8):708–12.
16. Zelickson B, Ross V, Kist D, et al. Ultrastructural effects of an infrared handpiece on forehead and abdominal skin. Dermatol Surg 2006;32(7):897–901.
17. Ruiz-Esparza J. Near painless, nonablative, immediate skin contraction induced by low-fluence irradiation with new infrared device: a report of 25 patients. Dermatol Surg 2006;32:601–10.
18. Alexiades-Armenakas M. Aging facial skin: lasers and related spectrum technologies. Facial Plast Surg Clin N Am 2011; 19(2):361–70.
19. Dierickx CC. The role of deep heating for noninvasive skin rejuvenation. Lasers Surg Med 2006;38(9):799–807.
20. Brightman L, Weiss E, Chapas AM, et al. Improvement in arm and post-partum abdominal and flank subcutaneous fat deposits and skin laxity using a bipolar radiofrequency, infrared, vacuum and mechanical massage device. Lasers Surg Med 2009;41(10): 791–8.
21. Tazi E, Alster TS. Noninvasive tissue tightening. In: Kaminer MS, Arndt KA, Dover JS, et al., editors. Atlas of cosmetic surgery. 2nd ed. Philadelphia: Elsevier; 2009. p. 209–23.
22. Taub AF, Battle EF Jr, Nikolaidis G. Multicenter clinical perspectives on a broadband infrared light device for skin tightening. J Drugs Dermatol 2006;5(8):771–8.
23. Alexiades-Armenakas M, Dover JS, Arndt KA. Unipolar versus bipolar radiofrequency treatment of rhytides and laxity using a mobile painless delivery method. Lasers Surg Med 2008;40(7): 446–53.
24. Blyumin-Karasik M, Rouhani P, Avashia N, et al. Skin tightening of aging upper arms using an infrared light device. Dermatol Surg 2011;37(4):441–9.
25. Felici M, Gentile P, De Angelis B, et al. The use of infrared radiation in the treatment of skin laxity. J Cosmet Laser Ther 2013;epub.
26. Winter ML. Post-pregnancy body contouring using a combined radiofrequency, infrared light and tissue manipulation device. J Cosmet Laser Ther 2009;11:229–35.
27. Narukar V. Full thickness permanent scars from bulk heating using an infrared light source. Lasers Surg Med 2006;S18:96.

Radiofrequency Treatment: Skin Tightening

3

Melissa A. Bogle, Michael S. Kaminer

Key Messages

- There is a high patient demand for safe and effective ways to decrease redundant or lax skin and smooth irregular body contours
- Patients tend to prefer noninvasive skin-tightening procedures with less risk, no scarring and reduced recovery time despite a decrease in effectiveness when compared with traditional skin excision techniques such as abdominoplasty or brachioplasty
- Treatment protocols with reduced energy settings are standard of care, increasing the safety profile and decreasing discomfort for the patient
- All radiofrequency skin-tightening devices work by a similar mechanism of action, which includes delivering heat in the form of energy to the skin or underlying structures and creating mechanical and biochemical effects that lead to both immediate collagen contraction and delayed remodeling and neocollagenesis due to the subsequent wound healing response
- Adjunctive treatment strategies can be used to increase patient satisfaction. Skin-tightening procedures on the body can be performed along with liposuction or other laser or light-based devices to address multiple issues and achieve improved overall results

Introduction

Skin laxity may result from chronological aging, photoaging, and changes in body dimensions during pregnancy or weight loss. Over the past decade, there has been increasing demand for safe and effective ways to decrease redundant or lax skin and smooth irregular body contours. Patients desire procedures with reduced recovery time, reduced risk and adequate clinical improvement. This has led to exponential growth in noninvasive body contouring and minimally invasive, nonablative tissue-tightening techniques, including laser, radiofrequency and ultrasound-based devices. The goal of this chapter is to review the use of radiofrequency devices in skin tightening specifically on the body.

Proposed mechanism(s) of action

Radiofrequency energy was the first modality specifically marketed for noninvasive skin tightening. Radiofrequency devices work by producing an alternating current that creates an electric field throughout the skin. The electric field shifts polarity millions of times per second, causing a change in the orientation of charged particles within the electric field. Heat is generated via tissue resistance to the movement of oscillating electrons within the radiofrequency field as governed by Ohm's law:

$$\text{Energy (joules)} = I^2 \times Z \times t$$
$$\text{where } I = \text{current (amps)}, Z = \text{impedance (ohms)}$$
$$\text{and } t = \text{time (seconds)}$$

The process does not follow the principles of selective photothermolysis as heat is generated by the skin's resistance to the flow of current within an electric field, rather than chromophore-based photon absorption as with a laser. This makes radiofrequency technologies well suited for deep dermal heating as opposed to light-based technologies which have a suboptimal depth potential due to energy being scattered or absorbed in the upper layers of the skin. The depth of energy delivered by a radiofrequency device depends on several factors, including the arrangement of radiofrequency electrodes (monopolar or bipolar), the type of tissue serving as the conduction medium (fat, skin), temperature, and the frequency of the electrical current applied.[1]

Radiofrequency energy is thought to induce skin tightening of the body by several mechanisms. The first is the immediate contraction of collagen fibers and fibrous septa in the subcutaneous fat due to direct thermal heating. Studies on samples of human abdominal skin have shown that when collagen fibers are heated to specific temperatures with radiofrequency energy, they contract due to breakage of intramolecular hydrogen bonds linking protein chains in the triple helix structure (denaturation). Contraction causes the helix to fold, leading to shorter, thicker, more 'compact' collagen fibers. Secondary wound healing also plays a role in tissue tightening with delayed

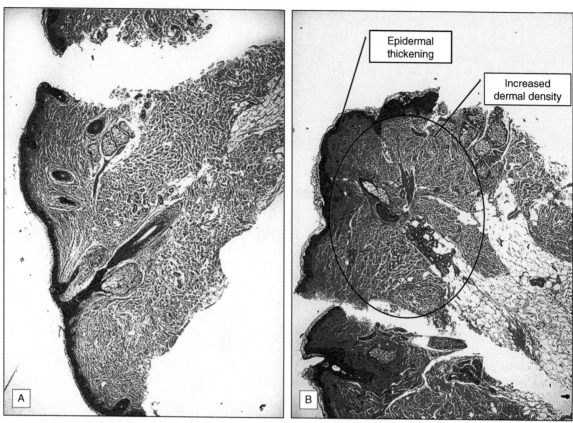

Figure 3.1 Human skin **(A)** before and **(B)** 4 months after treatment with the ThermaCool TC®, showing epidermal thickening as well as increased dermal density (*photograph courtesy of Thermage, Solta Medical, Inc.*)

remodeling and neocollagenesis over time (Fig. 3.1). It has been postulated that thermal heating by radiofrequency energy results in a microinflammatory stimulation of fibroblasts which induces new collagen and elastin as well as encouraging collagen reorganization into parallel arrays of compact fibrils.[2,3] Thus, radiofrequency effects are based on mild heating of the collagen and elastin fibers which can lead to collagen shrinkage and dermal thickening with a resulting improvement in firmness and elasticity of the skin. The degree of tissue tightening is dependent upon several factors, including the maximum temperature reached, the heat exposure time, tissue hydration, and tissue age.[4]

Patient selection

Radiofrequency energy differs from laser energy in that it does not depend on the principles of selective photothermolysis; therefore, radiofrequency procedures are appropriate for all skin types regardless of color. The exception is with combination devices that also have an optical component absorbed by pigment such as intense pulsed light. Such devices should be used with caution in patients with skin types IV–VI, over darkly pigmented lesions or areas

of dense pigment irregularity, or in lighter skin patients with a tan. Areas commonly treated with radiofrequency include the thighs, upper arms, abdomen, buttocks, and chest.

Pearl 1

Appropriate selection of patients and managing realistic expectations are key to ensuring patient satisfaction.

As with any other aesthetic procedure, appropriate selection of patients and managing realistic expectations are key to ensuring patient satisfaction. Patients must be advised that it takes time to see maximal improvement and that final results occur over a period of 3–6 months. The most appropriate candidates are those who are younger with mild or mild to moderate skin laxity.

Pearl 2

The most appropriate candidates for radiofrequency skin tightening of the body are those who have mild or mild to moderate skin laxity without underlying structural ptosis.

Younger patients are thought to respond better than older patients because heat-labile collagen bonds are progressively replaced by irreducible multivalent cross-links as tissue ages, such that the skin of older individuals is more resistant to heat-induced tissue tightening.[5] Skin quality, however, is more important than the absolute age of the patient. Older patients with good skin quality can generally be expected to have a promising response to therapy. Individuals with severe skin laxity will achieve a more dramatic outcome with a surgical skin excision, such as an abdominoplasty or brachioplasty, if they are willing to accept the risks, recovery time, and resulting scars associated with traditional surgical approaches. The benefits, risks, and limitations of the various types of radiofrequency devices should be discussed with the patient in detail, including a mention of alternative therapies so that the patient can make an informed decision.

Pearl 3

Younger patients may respond better than older patients; however, older patients with good overall skin quality may respond just as well as their younger counterparts.

The ideal patient should also have primarily skin laxity without underlying structural ptosis or other contributing issues. This is of particular importance with skin-tightening procedures on the abdomen where muscular problems, such as diastasis recti post-pregnancy, can contribute to a lax appearance and will not be addressed through radiofrequency skin tightening. Patients should also understand that radiofrequency alone is not effective for the superficial textural and pigmentary aspects of photoaging such as wrinkles, lentigines, and telangiectases.

Contraindications to the use of radiofrequency procedures include pregnancy, active collagen vascular disorders, any implanted electrical device such as pacemakers or internal defibrillators, and the presence of any metallic device (i.e. hip replacement, hip or femur surgery).

Typical treatment course

Radiofrequency skin-tightening treatments are performed in the office on an outpatient basis. Individual patient pain feedback should be used as a basis for energy selection in a given treatment area. Anesthesia is usually not required with current treatment protocols, although topical anesthetic may be used if warranted. Some authors have suggested topical anesthetics are not helpful in alleviating deep dermal heat sensations and may actually exacerbate discomfort by selectively numbing the epidermis so that the patient does not feel the cooling relief of technologies that use cryogen spray cooling when the tip is in contact with the skin.[6] The use of oral analgesics, nerve blocks, or intravenous sedation should not be used because pain feedback from the patient is necessary to limit side effects and enhance patient safety. Local infiltration anesthesia is

also not recommended as the fluid may alter the tissue conductivity and increase the risk of adverse events.

It is essential to take standardized pre-procedure photographs before each treatment. The photographer should be careful to use identical positioning and lighting conditions in each session, as subtle differences may distort patient perceptions. Pre-treatment photographs may need to be compared with post-treatment photographs as changes with radiofrequency procedures may be mild, evolve over 3 to 6 months, and may go unnoticed by the patient.

Pearl 4

Patient pain feedback should be used as the basis for choosing particular energies in a given treatment area for each individual. This will help to limit side effects, enhance patient safety, and maximize results.

Patients should be asked throughout the treatment about their level of pain on a scale of 1 to 10. The goal is to calibrate temperature settings to keep the pain level below a 5 or 6. High pain levels mean the temperature is too great and should be turned down to reduce the risk of adverse events. Persistent erythema, localized swelling or hives are all indicators that the tissue has not had sufficient time to cool before additional passes may be considered. The number of treatments varies depending on the device, treatment parameters, area of the body, degree of skin laxity, and individual patient response.

A considerable array of radiofrequency devices is available for clinical use (Table 3.1). They may be broadly categorized by the arrangement of electrodes as either monopolar, bipolar, or unipolar.[7] The various systems create different electromagnetic fields. However, the interaction of the energy with the target tissue is similar (Fig. 3.2). In a monopolar system, the skin tightening effect is based on the principle of uniform volumetric heating. Electrical current is delivered via a single electrode in the handpiece in contact with the skin, exiting to a grounding pad. Without appropriate surface cooling,

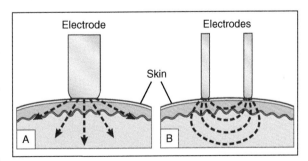

Figure 3.2 (A) In a monopolar electrode system, current is delivered via a single electrode in the handpiece in contact with the skin. **(B)** In a bipolar electrode system, current passes between two electrodes within the handpiece at a fixed distance over the skin

Table 3.1 Devices for skin tightening and body contouring

Product/device	Manufacturer	Frequency	Output energy	Delivery system	Features
Monopolar devices					
Exilis	BTL Aesthetics, Prague, CR	3.4 MHz	Up to 120 W/90 W		Monopolar energy flow control, safety system, built-in thermometer, no risk of overheating
Thermage®	Solta Medical, Hayward, CA	6.78 MHz	400 W		New handpiece (CPT: comfortable pulse technology) with vibrations to improve patient comfort. Pain nerval interceptors get confused and busy (vibrations, cooling, heating)
Cutera®	TruSculpt, Brisbane, CA	1 MHz	N/A		Handpiece that reads out once optimal temperature of 43–45 °C is reached
Ellman®	Pellevue, Oceanside, NY	4 MHz alternating	Levels		Several handpieces for smaller areas. Can also use unit as an electrocautery unit
Biorad	GSD Tech Co., Shenzhen, China	1.15 MHz	1000 W max		Continuous cooling; automatic resistance technology, single and continuous mode
Bipolar devices					
Accent Family	Alma Lasers, Caesarea, Israel	40.68 MHz	Up to 300 W	Multiple devices	Unipolar, bipolar, fractionated
VelaShape II™	Syneron/Candela, San Jose, CA	N/A	Infrared – up to 35 W RF – up to 60 W	Handpiece w/bipolar radiofrequency, infrared laser, suction	Vsmooth (40 × 40 mm) and Vcontour (30 × 30 mm) treatment areas
eMatrix		N/A	Up to 62 mJ/min	Matrix of electrodes	Disposable tip
TriPollar™ Apollo®	Pollogen, Tel Aviv, Israel	1 MHz	50 W	3 handpieces	Large, medium, small
Reaction™	Viora, Jersey City, NJ	0.8, 1.7, 2.45, MHz	Body 50 W, face 20 W	4 modes: 0.8, 1.7, 2.45 + multichannel	SVC (suction, vacuum cooling)
V-Touch™	Viora, Jersey City, NJ	N/A	N/A	3 handpieces: 0.8, 1.7, 2.45	SVC (suction, vacuum cooling)
EndyMed™ PRO 3DEEP 3 Pole	EndyMed Medical, Caesarea, Israel	1 MHz	65 W	4 handpieces	3 deep RF handpieces: skin tightening, body contouring, facial tightening, fractional skin resurfacing
Venus Concept-8 Circular Poles	Venus Freeze, Toronto, ON	RF: 1 MHz Magnetic pulse: 1.5 Hz	RF: up to 150 W Magnetic flux: 15 Gauss	Large handpiece 8 poles 5 mm apart, dual mode = bipolar + magnetic field	Multipolar RF and magnetic pulse
TiteFX	Invasix, Yokeneam, Israel	1 MHz	60 W	Bi-RF + vacuum	Bipolar w/suction real time epidermal temperature monitor

Table 3.1   Devices for skin tightening and body contouring—cont'd

Product/device	Manufacturer	Frequency	Output energy	Delivery system	Features
Aurora SR	Syneron/Candela, San Jose, CA	–	Up to 25 J/cm^3	400–980 nm 580–980 nm 680–980 nm	RF and IPL (intense pulsed light)
VelaSmooth™	Syneron/Candela, San Jose, CA	–	700–200 nm	Handpiece	RF/infrared light with mechanical manipulation
Aluma™	Lumenis Ltd, Yokneam, Israel	40.68 MHz	Up to 300 W	Bipolar and UniLarge handpieces	FACES technology using functional aspiration
ePrime	Syneron/Candela, San Jose, CA	460 ± 5 kHz	84 VRMS	Microneedles	20° delivery angle, injected into dermis
eTwo	Syneron/Candela, San Jose, CA	–	62 mJ sublative; 100 J/cm^3 sublime	Matrix of electrodes	RF/infrared light
elos Plus	Syneron/Candela, San Jose, CA	1–3 Hz	Variable	8 different applicators	RF/infrared light
Unipolar series					
Accent® RF	Alma Lasers, Caesarea, Israel	40.68 MHz	Up to 200 W	1 handpiece	Unipolar energy to heat fat, bipolar to deliver energy to dermis
Vanquish	BTL Aesthetics, Prague, Czech Republic	–	–	Non-contact	Operator independent

Adapted from Beasley KL, Weiss RA. Radiofrequency in cosmetic dermatology. Dermatol Clin 2004;32:79–90, with permission.

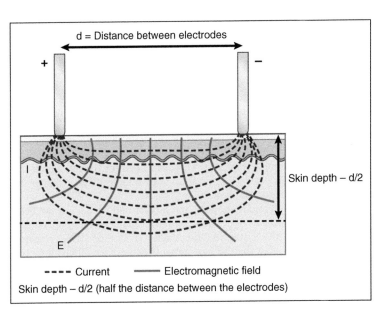

d = Distance between electrodes

Skin depth – d/2

- - - - Current   ——— Electromagnetic field

Skin depth – d/2 (half the distance between the electrodes)

Figure 3.3 In a bipolar electrode system, the penetration depth of energy into the tissue is approximately half the distance between the two electrodes

there may be a high density of power close to the electrode's surface which may lead to safety concerns such as burns or overheating.[1,8] In a bipolar system, the electrical current passes between two electrodes within the handpiece at a fixed distance over the skin. The advantage of bipolar systems is a more controlled current distribution. The disadvantage is that the penetration depth of energy into tissue is limited to roughly half the distance between the electrodes (Fig. 3.3).[1,8] With a unipolar radiofrequency system there is one electrode, no grounding pad, and a large radiofrequency field emitted in an omnidirectional field around the electrode, similar to that of a radio antenna.[7]

Electrical conductivity varies among different types of tissue, between individual patients, and under different operating conditions. Even under otherwise equal treatment parameters, not all patients will have the same amount of energy deposited in a particular area. This is because each individual patient has a unique tissue structure with varying dermal thickness, fat thickness, fibrous septa, and number and size of adnexal structures, all of which play a role in determining impedance and heat perception.[1,9,10] In general, fat, bone and dry skin tend to have lower conductivities so current tends to flow around those structures rather than passing through them. Wet skin has a higher electrical conductivity than dry skin, so increasing skin hydration with generous amounts of coupling fluid can increase results in certain radiofrequency procedures.[1]

Temperature also influences tissue conductivity. The distribution of electrical current within the skin may be influenced by pre-heating or cooling selected targets within the field.[1] Pre-heating a target such as a hair or vessel with light energy will, in theory, decrease resistance and increase conductivity of the radiofrequency current in that area making it possible to selectively increase the amount of radiofrequency energy that reaches a particular target. Conversely, surface cooling increases resistance to the electrical field near the epidermis such that the current is driven deeper into the skin and the depth of penetration is increased.[1]

Numerous device variations exist, combining radiofrequency technology with additions such as laser or intense pulsed light, fractional delivery, electrodes inserted into the skin, vacuum suction, and vibration and/or massage.

Expected outcomes

In terms of expectations, nonablative skin-tightening technologies should not be thought of as equivalent to traditional surgical lifting, but as an alternative option for a subset of patients who either have a modest amount of skin laxity or who are willing to trade a dramatic improvement for minimal risk and recovery time. Despite a number of clinical studies reporting significant improvement in the appearance of skin laxity, clinical results are generally mild and a small number of patients may perceive no improvement at all.[11]

In 2004 Zelickson and colleagues evaluated the effects of monopolar radiofrequency on human abdominal skin at treatment energies ranging from 95 to 181 J.[2] Treatment effects were analyzed by both light and electron microscopy of punch biopsies taken immediately after and up to 8 weeks post-treatment. They found a mild perivascular and perifollicular inflammatory infiltrate immediately post-procedure along with collagen fibers that were shorter and thicker than baseline at 0, 3, and 8 weeks post-treatment. Changes were observed up to a skin depth

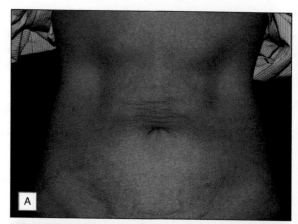

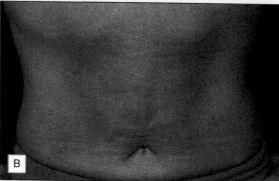

Figure 3.4 Tightening of abdominal skin with the ThermaCool TC® (Solta Medical, Inc). **(A)** Pre-treatment. **(B)** 1 year after treatment, one pass at 15.5 J

of approximately 5 mm indicating mid to deep dermis (Fig. 3.4).[2]

Unfortunately, the majority of clinical studies evaluating radiofrequency energy for skin tightening have been done on the head and neck. Most studies looking at radiofrequency treatments on the body have focused on cellulite reduction or fat layer reduction as the clinical endpoint (Fig. 3.5). There is a need for further controlled trials evaluating the success of radiofrequency skin tightening on the body.

Hybrid monopolar and bipolar radiofrequency has been investigated for body contouring and treatment of cellulite on the buttocks and thighs (Fig. 3.6). This research revealed that 68% of patients achieved a 20% volumetric reduction of the fat layer (determined by ultrasound) after two treatment sessions, indicating contraction of the subcutaneous adipose tissue.[12]

A study designed to evaluate the use of a bipolar radiofrequency device combined with infrared, vacuum and mechanical massage for skin laxity of the arms and abdomen in 19 subjects with four to five weekly treatments revealed a statistically significant change in arm circumference after five treatments (mean loss of 0.625 cm) and a statistically significant change in

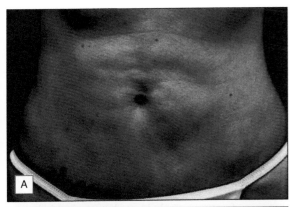

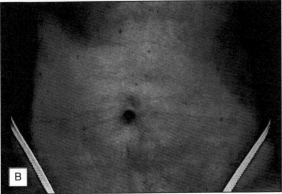

Figure 3.5 Skin tightening of the abdomen in addition to reduction of excess fat and cellulite **(A)** before, and **(B)** after seven treatments with the VelaShape device (Syneron-Candela) *(from Sadick NS. VelaSmooth and VelaShape. In: Goldman MP, Hexsel D, editors. Cellulite: pathophysiology and treatment. 2nd ed. New York: Informa Healthcare, 2010. p. 108–14, with permission)*

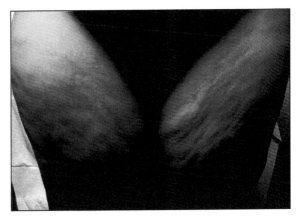

Figure 3.6 Unilateral treatment showing skin tightening and reduction of cellulite on the right leg following five treatments with the Accent device (Alma Lasers), the left leg serving as an untreated control *(courtesy of Dr. Macrene Alexiades-Armenakas)*

abdominal circumference after three treatments (mean loss of 1.25 cm).[13]

In 2012, a group treated 16 women with a bipolar radiofrequency device combined with a mechanical massage technique for moderate to severe wrinkles and/or lax, sagging skin on the face and body with three treatment sessions at 3-week intervals. Those who underwent body treatments were treated only on the right side of the body, with the left side serving as an untreated control. 50% of patients demonstrated moderate improvement (51–75%) and 31% of patients demonstrated significant improvement (>75%).[4]

Additional research is also required to compare the various radiofrequency devices to determine whether there are any particular advantages of one over another. One report has suggested a hybrid monopolar and bipolar radiofrequency device may be a better choice for tissue tightening and volume reduction on the body.[14] The report compared treatment of one arm with a monopolar radiofrequency device and the opposite arm with a hybrid monopolar and bipolar radiofrequency device. The monopolar radiofrequency arm was treated with a single treatment at settings of 351.5 to 354 with a minimum of

six passes on the inner arm and three passes on the outer arm (1200 pulses total). The hybrid arm was treated with a series of nine treatments at 2-week intervals using the monopolar handpiece at an epidermal temperature of 42.5 °C with three therapeutic phase passes. Skin texture improved with both treatments; however, the hybrid treated arm was reported to be tighter and firmer after just two treatments, with a looser-fitting clothing sleeve. Each hybrid treatment took approximately 30 minutes while the monopolar radiofrequency treatment took approximately 2 hours. While continued improvement may have been seen with multiple treatments with the monopolar radiofrequency device, the author suggests that this would not have been cost or time effective due to the expensive consumables and long treatment times.[14] The monopolar-treated arm did not have a looser-fitting clothing sleeve until the physician had returned at the end of the study and performed two additional hybrid treatments, leading the author to suggest that the hybrid monopolar and bipolar radiofrequency energy device penetrates deeper and may be the device of choice when patients require both tissue tightening and volume reduction.[14]

Long-term studies to examine the longevity of radiofrequency-induced skin tightening have not been performed, but it appears that patients can at least expect a period of a year or more before touch-up treatments are required.

Safety

The most common potential problems with radiofrequency skin tightening are pain during the procedure, temporary surface irregularities, post-treatment changes in sensation, and unrealistic patient expectations. Low energy, multiple pass protocols are significantly safer than the original high energy protocols with monopolar radiofrequency, lowering the incidence of adverse events to less than 0.05% from the previous incidence of less than 1%.[15] The majority of side effects were seen in the early years of the use of radiofrequency for skin tightening when treatment protocols were initially being established.

Pearl 5

Most skin-tightening treatments using radiofrequency, ultrasound and infrared light are generally safe in all skin types. The exception is technologies that use an optical component absorbed by pigment, such as the intense pulsed light–radiofrequency combination device.

Surface irregularities can include small nodules or lumps that patients feel but rarely see on casual inspection as well as indentations. The latter are most common with treatment over thin-skinned areas and typically self-resolve within a few weeks. Depressions or indentations are thought to be due to excessive heating of the fat lobules and fibrous septa. The incidence is rare with current treatment protocols and current generation treatment tips. Changes in sensation may include itching, tingling or temporary numbness. Symptoms are usually mild and resolve completely in days to weeks.

Side effects related to overly aggressive treatment include burns, blisters, crusting, indentations, scars or changes in pigmentation (hyper- or hypopigmentation). The overall incidence of such problems is rare and unlikely to occur with the use of current standard of care treatment protocols involving patient pain feedback to guide parameter selection. Patients should be carefully inspected post-procedure for signs of overheating or a heightened inflammatory response in the treatment area such as whitening, persistent erythema, localized swelling, or hives. If any of these indications are found, it may be helpful to ice the area and apply a mid- to high-potency topical corticosteroid cream to help decrease the risk of crusting or pigment alteration.

Multi-modality approaches

Combination therapy is a well-established approach in cosmetic dermatology to help provide optimal outcomes with decreased risk. Patients wishing to undergo noninvasive skin tightening on the body may achieve best results when radiofrequency treatments are done in combination with other procedures geared toward fat reduction, body shaping, or improving the surface texture and appearance of the skin itself. Patients may perceive an overall lack of skin 'tone' in an area, which is an ill-defined complaint that may have several contributing factors, including loss of collagen and elasticity, increased skin laxity, and irregularities in surface color or texture. For example, a patient who is bothered by crêpey, 'cigarette paper' skin on the arms, chest, abdomen or thighs in addition to redundant skin would benefit from fractional resurfacing procedures in combination with radiofrequency skin tightening to best address the surface changes as well as the loss of collagen and elasticity in the deeper dermis.

In addition, cumulative effectiveness may sometimes be increased by combining liposuction with radiofrequency procedures in areas such as the abdomen and back of the arms.[4] Radiofrequency procedures should not be performed for at least 2 weeks after administration of tumescent anesthesia as the tumescent solution may influence tissue conductivity and the patient's pain feedback response will not be a reliable indicator for selection of treatment parameters.

Conclusion

The quest for nonsurgical skin tightening has led to an increasing number of devices on the market. Radiofrequency skin tightening applications on the body appear best suited for younger patients with mild to moderate skin laxity without a significant degree of underlying structural contributions. The key to success is patient selection, management of expectations, and adherence to conservative treatment protocols. Future research and clinical trials will continue to refine techniques and delivery systems for optimal results.

CASE STUDY 1

A 36-year-old woman presents to your office for a consultation regarding her abdomen. She has had three children and states that she follows a healthy diet and works out 5 days per week in the gym with a combination of strength training and aerobic activity. She feels that no matter how much she works out, she just cannot tone her abdomen and wants to look her best for a beach vacation she and her husband have planned for their 10th wedding anniversary next year. She is wondering specifically about liposuction. She states that she does not expect perfection, but just wants to look as good as she possibly can. On examination, the patient is thin and fit with mild excess skin laxity localized to the abdomen. A 'pinch test' of the abdominal bulge is less than a finger width in diameter, indicating predominantly skin laxity with little subcutaneous fat. You find no evidence of underlying diastasis or separation of the rectus abdominis muscles when the abdomen is palpated as the patient contracts her abdominal muscles. This patient is an ideal candidate for radiofrequency skin tightening of the abdomen. She is not an appropriate candidate for liposuction as she is very thin with little subcutaneous fat. Liposuction would run the risk of contour irregularities and dimpling. The patient also has appropriate expectations, is in a younger age category, and does not have contributing underlying structural issues that need to be surgically addressed. Although surgical abdominoplasty is an alternative option, the patient's skin laxity is mild and the risks, resulting scar and recovery process may not be worth the benefit in this case. Her goal is to look good for a beach vacation in 1 year. This gives plenty of time to obtain maximal results due to the delayed wound healing process and even allows time for multiple treatments if needed.

CASE STUDY 2

A 72-year-old female presents for a consultation to improve what she calls her 'bat wing' arms. She had a brachioplasty 5 years ago and states that helped immensely, but she is still bothered by her arms and only wears long sleeves. She feels that the skin on the arms is 'jiggly', particularly posteriorly. She would like further improvement but does not want to undergo surgery again as she feels it took several years for the scars to 'settle down'. Her goal is to be able to wear short-sleeve or sleeveless tops without feeling self-conscious. She follows a healthy diet but has difficulty finding time to regularly exercise. On examination, the patient has excess skin laxity on the upper arms, with a mild to moderate bat-wing deformity despite her previous brachioplasty procedure and a moderate degree of subcutaneous fat. There is a well-healed, faded scar extending from her axilla to the elbow. The patient has significant photodamage with thin, crêpey skin. This patient has several options for improvement of her upper arms. She could undergo a second brachioplasty procedure using the existing scars to hide the new excisions. She was happy with her previous results; however, she does not wish to undergo surgery again due to the prolonged recovery time. Given this factor, she would be a good candidate for a combination procedure involving liposuction (or noninvasive fat removal with radiofrequency, ultrasound, or cryolipolysis) of the upper arms followed by radiofrequency skin tightening. Due to her age, poor skin quality, and degree of skin laxity, radiofrequency skin tightening alone may not give her enough of a result to match her expectations. By performing the radiofrequency procedure sequentially following fat removal, the patient would likely get more improvement than with either procedure alone. For best results, it would be ideal to also address the patient's thin, crêpey skin texture on the upper arms with a series of fractional resurfacing treatments if she is willing to undergo further procedures and it falls within her budget.

References

1. Bogle MA. Radiofrequency energy and hybrid devices. In: Alam M, Dover JS, editors. Procedures in Cosmetic Dermatology Series: Non-surgical skin tightening and lifting. Philadelphia: WB Saunders; 2008. p. 21–32.
2. Zelickson B, Kist D, Bernstein E, et al. Histological and ultrastructural evaluation of the effects of a radiofrequency-based nonablative dermal remodeling device: a pilot study. Arch Dermatol 2004;140:204–9.
3. Hantash BM, Ubeid AA, Chang H, et al. Bipolar fractional radiofrequency treatment induces neoelastogenesis and neocollagenesis. Lasers Surg Med 2009;41:1–9.
4. Belensky I, Margulis A, Elman M, et al. Exploring channeling optimized radiofrequency energy: a review of radiofrequency history and applications in esthetic fields. Adv Ther 2012;29:249–66.
5. Hsu TS, Kaminer MS. The use of nonablative radiofrequency technology to tighten the lower face and neck. Semin Cutan Med Surg 2003;22:115–23.
6. Dierickx CC. The role of deep heating for noninvasive skin rejuvenation. Lasers Surg Med 2006;38:799–807.
7. Beasley KL, Weiss RA. Radiofrequency in cosmetic dermatology. Dermatol Clin 2014;32:79–90.
8. Gold MH, Goldman MP, Rao J, et al. Treatment of wrinkles and elastosis using vacuum-assisted bipolar radiofrequency heating of the dermis. Dermatol Surg 2007;33:300–9.
9. Abraham MT, Ross EV. Current concepts in nonablative radiofrequency rejuvenation of the lower face and neck. Facial Plast Surg 2005;21:65–73.
10. Lack EB, Rachel JD, D'Andrea L, Corres J. Relationship of energy settings and impedance in different anatomic areas using a radiofrequency device. Dermatol Surg 2005;31:1668–70.
11. Bogle MA, Uebelhoer N, Weiss RA, Mayoral F. Evaluation of the multiple pass, low fluence algorithm for radiofrequency tightening of the lower face. Lasers Surg Med 2007;39:210–17.
12. Del Pino E, Rosado RH, Azuela A, et al. Effect of controlled volumetric tissue heating with radiofrequency on cellulite and the subcutaneous tissue of the buttocks and thighs. J Drugs Dermatol 2006;5:714–22.
13. Brightman L, Weiss E, Chapas AM, et al. Improvement in arm and post-partum abdominal and flank subcutaneous fat deposits and skin laxity using a bipolar radiofrequency, infrared, vacuum and mechanical massage device. Lasers Surg Med 2009;41:791–8.
14. Mayoral FA. Skin tightening with a combined unipolar and bipolar radiofrequency device. J Drugs Dermatol 2007;6:212–15.
15. Narins RS, Tope WD, Pope K, Ross E. Overtreatment effects associated with a radiofrequency tissue-tightening device: rare, preventable, and correctable with subcision and autologous fat transfer. Dermatol Surg 2006;32:115–24.

Micro-focused Ultrasound: Skin Tightening

4

Kira Minkis, George J. Hruza, Murad Alam

Key Messages

- Skin laxity is a common sign of photoaging
- Skin lifting and tightening are desirable outcomes for a large majority of patients interested in photo-rejuvenation
- Noninvasive treatment options for skin tightening and skin lifting are very limited.
- Micro-focused ultrasound with visualization (MFU-V) has been shown to provide skin lifting and tightening, making it the only FDA cleared technology (Ulthera Inc., Mesa, AZ) with a 'lifting' indication
- MFU-V is a safe and efficacious treatment for mild to moderate laxity

Introduction

Skin tightening and lifting continues to be a sought-after goal for millions of people across the globe. Despite much in the way of advances in our ability to improve and enhance various aspects of photoaging, until recently our capacity for safe and effective skin tightening has been limited. Photoaging occurs in a semi-predictable stepwise progression which includes both textural as well as pigmentary alterations to the skin. In the initial steps of skin aging, dynamic rhytides are evident in areas of skin movement and these eventuate into static rhytides. With further aging, the skin begins to develop laxity, which is often most evident in the jowls and submental skin. Photo-rejuvenation of the skin, in its optimum, should address all of these components of aging skin. Traditionally, various energy delivery devices have been used to treat several components of skin aging, including rhytides, laxity, and dyschromia, such as ablative CO_2 or Er:YAG laser devices, as well as treatments such as deep chemical peels and dermabrasion. These methods relied on ablation of the epidermis causing re-epithelialization while delivering significant thermal injury to the dermis sufficient to stimulate a robust wound healing response with subsequent collagen remodeling and contraction leading to decreased rhytides, improvement in skin texture, skin tightening and lifting, and improvement in pigmentation. However, despite significant improvement in these skin characteristics and efficacy of these treatments, significant patient downtime, long and painful post-treatment healing and substantial side effects were major drawbacks of these ablative procedures.

In recent years, multiple treatment modalities have become available for treatment of skin wrinkling and laxity in a nonablative manner. These include lasers and light devices, infrared energy devices as well as energy-based procedures including radiofrequency with and without ablation. These allow the use of thermal energy to target the reticular dermis and subcutis in an effort to cause tissue contraction and dermal remodeling whilst minimizing undesirable epidermal injury. As a result, 'downtime' is minimized with expedient post-procedure healing allowing the patient to proceed with their regular activities shortly after treatment and minimizing the necessity to interrupt a busy patient's work or social schedule. Additionally, minimal epidermal injury allows for safer treatment among a wider range of skin types and reduces the risk of adverse events compared to either ablative resurfacing or more invasive surgical procedures such as rhytidectomy. However, the drawback of these safer nonablative methods is that, relative to their invasive and ablative counterparts, the results are often modest, less reliable, and result in an inconsistent duration of benefit. Individual variation in responsiveness to noninvasive skin tightening has also been significant. Ultrasound (US) is an energy modality that can be focused in the skin and subcutis to cause thermal coagulation at specific desired depths, while also allowing for real-time visualization of tissue targets for energy deposition. Micro-focused US with visualization (MFU-V) for skin rejuvenation has been shown in recent studies to be safe and effective for skin lifting and tightening.

Pearl 1

MFU-V delivers energy to selected foci within the dermis and subcutis leading to the generation of heat and selective coagulative changes.

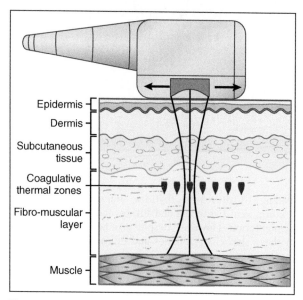

Figure 4.1 Ultrasound device applied to skin

MFU-V delivers inducible energy to selected foci within the dermis and subcutis leading to the generation of heat and selective coagulative changes (Fig. 4.1). The generated heat causes initiation of a tissue injury and repair cascade, the end result of which is a tightening of the skin. Results from several studies have led the currently available MFU-V device on the market, the Ulthera system (Fig. 4.2), to receive the first Food and Drug Administration (FDA) approval for skin lifting, initially for eyebrow lifting in 2009, followed by an approval for lifting the submentum and neck tissue in 2012. An advantage associated with this device is that the built-in diagnostic ultrasound may potentially improve targeting and hence safety (Fig. 4.3). Unfocused US energy can be used to image the treatment area while focused US energy can induce thermal injury of the mid to deep reticular dermis. Visualization of key structures with the diagnostic US can help ensure that the energy from the therapeutic device is delivered at the optimal points, and anatomic structures that do not need to be treated are spared.

The MFU-V device has been proven effective for the treatment of patients with mild to moderate laxity of the skin. Recently it has also been used in various other locations and applications, including tightening of the skin of the buttocks, décolleté, knees, and elbows, as well as for the treatment of acne and hyperhidrosis.

Proposed mechanism(s) of action

US includes the sound wave frequencies above the range of human hearing (18–20 kHz), and the Ulthera device operates at 4–10 MHz. US imaging is adapted to the visualization of the first 8 mm of tissue, thus specifically allowing for imaging of skin (see Fig. 4.3). The dual modality US device offered the capability of real-time imaging,

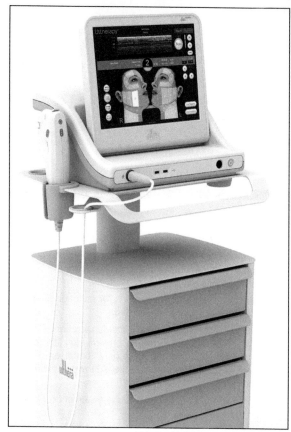

Figure 4.2 Ulthera MFU-V device *(from Ulthera Inc., Mesa, AZ, with permission)*

which allows visualization below the skin's surface as precisely-placed 'thermal coagulation points' (TCPs) are placed at prescribed depths. The resulting small micro-coagulation zones, approximately 1 mm^3 in size, cause thermal contraction of tissue. Subsequent wound healing results in neocollagenesis and collagen remodeling. A recent study using a safe nontoxic stable isotope (deuterated water) to quantitatively measure new collagen synthesis in vivo over a 4-week period following MFU-V treatment demonstrated that type I and type III collagen synthesis was increased by an average of 8.4% and 16.4%, respectively, when compared with control untreated tissue.[1]

Pearl 2

The generated heat causes initiation of the tissue repair cascade in which the end result is a tightening effect of the skin.

The Ulthera device consists of a central computerized power unit, a handpiece, and interchangeable transducers designed to target specific layers of the dermis and subcutis (see Fig. 4.2). The handpiece contains the transducer

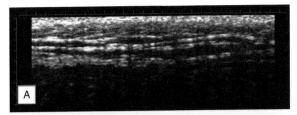

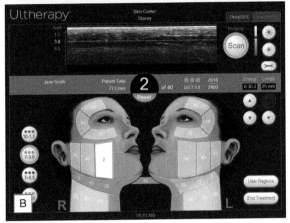

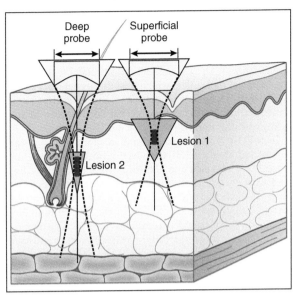

Figure 4.4 Zones of shallow and deep transducers creating triangular zones of thermal coagulation but at different depths in the dermis *(adapted from Alam et al. 2010, with permission)*.

Figure 4.3 (A) Sample ultrasound image prior to treatment. **(B)** The ultrasound image allows visualization of the different tissue planes, with the ultrasound focus (represented by the lines in the image) on the superficial musculo-aponeurotic system *(from Ulthera Inc., Mesa, AZ, with permission)*.

that enables sequential imaging (unfocused US energy, allowing visualization of dermal and subcutaneous structures) and treatment (delivery of focused US energy to create thermal injuries at specific depths in the skin).

The device initially had three transducers: 1) superficial: 7 MHz, 3.0 mm focus depth; 2) intermediate: 7 MHz, 4.5 mm focus depth; and 3) deep: 4 MHz, 4.5 mm focus depth. Most recently, a 10 MHz transducer capable of producing focal TCPs at depths of 1.5 mm into the dermis was introduced to induce more superficial dermal neocollagenesis. Human cadaveric tissues have demonstrated that penetration depth is determined by frequency, such that higher frequency waves produce a shallow focal injury zone and lower frequency waves have a greater depth of penetration to produce TCPs at deeper layers.[2]

Each transducer delivers US energy in a straight 25 mm line with spacing between each TCP of 1.1 mm for the 1.5 mm and 3.0 mm depths, and 1.5 mm for the 4.5 mm depths. Short pulse durations (25–50 ms) and relatively low energy (in the 0.20–1.2 J range), depending on the particular transducer, confine the TCPs to their target depth (Fig. 4.4). The handpiece is advanced in a line pattern at the set conditions (power, duration) and at the selective variables (length of treatment, spacing of exposures) to produce uniform tissue exposures for each 'line' of MFU-V treatment. Human cadaveric studies, as well as preclinical studies in porcine skin and pre-rhytidectomy excision skin, have confirmed consistency in the depth,

size, and orientation of TCP created by MFU-V in the subdermal soft tissue and deeper superficial musculo-aponeurotic system (SMAS) layers, with preservation of immediately adjacent soft tissue and structures.[3–6]

Thermal injury is confined by keeping the pulse duration relatively short. Provided that the energy delivered is not excessive for the focal depth and frequency emitted by a given transducer, the epidermal surface remains unaffected. Therefore, the need for epidermal cooling is eliminated.[4,5] Since the tissue is altered by arrays of small zones of focal damage rather than ablation of an entire macroscopic area, rapid healing occurs from tissue immediately adjacent to the thermal lesions. This is somewhat analogous to fractional laser ablation, except MFU-V affects only the deep dermal and subcutaneous tissue, as per the transducer selected, and the thermal injury zones are wider.

The lifting and tightening effect of US treatment is based on coagulative heating of specific zones of the dermis and subcutaneous tissue. The US energy is microfocused, such that thermal coagulation occurs only where the sound waves meet at discrete separated TCPs (see Figs 4.1 and 4.4). The size of the points varies based on the specific frequency and power settings used. This eventuates into nonsurgical tissue lifting without affecting the surface of the skin, thus making this technology safe to apply in all Fitzpatrick skin types with exceedingly low risk of hyper- or hypopigmentation. Apart from ionizing radiation, US is the only type of inducible energy that can be delivered arbitrarily deeply into tissue in a selective manner. The treatment is programmable for various depths and spacing based on transducer selection. Variability of energy delivery can occur in the actual treatment if there is improper skin contact, poor coupling, or too much pressure applied to the handpiece. Transcutaneous application of US into whole-organ soft tissue produces coagulative necrosis resulting primarily from thermal mechanisms.[7-9] The US field vibrates tissue, creating friction between molecules, which absorb mechanical energy that leads to secondary generation of heat. Selective coagulative change is affected within the focal region of the beam, with the immediately adjacent tissue spared.[3-6]

In MFU-V, energy is deposited in short pulses in the millisecond domain (50–200 ms). Avoiding cavitational processes, a frequency in the megahertz (MHz) range is used with energy levels deposited at each treatment site being on the order of 0.20–1.2 J. It is estimated that the device heats tissue to 65 °C–70 °C, the critical temperature at which collagen denaturation occurs with instigation of the tissue repair cascade. Precise microcoagulation points deep in the dermis as well as the SMAS have been demonstrated.[4,8] Suh et al.[10] demonstrate histologic evidence that both dermal collagen and elastic fibers are significantly regenerated and increase in number, resulting in thickening of the reticular dermis with no significant change in the epidermis. These authors conclude that it is via this dermal collagen regeneration that the rejuvenation of infraorbital laxity is achieved. This effect of increasing collagen synthesis has recently been quantitatively measured after treatment.

Microcoagulation is thought to cause gradual tightening of the skin through collagen contraction and remodeling. The initial collagen denaturation is followed by gradual tissue contraction over approximately 3 months. The duration of clinical lifting response is permanent but as patients continue to age, new collagen breaks down as part of the aging process. No controlled studies have thus far been performed to evaluate the clinical response relative to other similar skin-tightening treatments with radiofrequency or laser energy sources.

Patient selection

Good candidates are patients who wish to avoid a surgical facelift but who would like treatment of skin laxity. The ideal patient for nonsurgical tissue tightening displays mild to moderate skin and soft tissue laxity. Preferably, patients should be nonsmokers, not obese, and ideal candidates should not have excessive sagging or photoaging as their ability to create collagen in response to thermal injury may be inadequate.

Pearl 3

The ideal patient for nonsurgical tissue tightening displays mild to moderate skin and soft tissue laxity.

Severe aging, tissue heaviness and fullness also negatively impact results as they may impede the lifting effects after thermally induced collagen shortening and stimulation of new collagen synthesis.

MFU-V appears safe across all skin types. Suh et al.[11] were the first to demonstrate safety and efficacy of MFU-V in Asian skin (Fitzpatrick skin types III–VI). The few absolute contraindications include open skin at the treatment site, severe or active cystic acne, and implanted pacemakers and cardiac devices in the area. Relative contraindications include medical conditions and/or medications that alter or impair wound healing.

Setting realistic patient expectations is of paramount importance prior to treatment. It is helpful to obtain good photographs before and after treatment. Pre-operative consultation may also include a detailed discussion of areas that are most problematic for the patient, expected results, limitations, and the potential for no appreciable clinical improvement.

Typical treatment course

The depth of treatment, and therefore the selection of the transducer, is dictated by the thickness of the skin at the treatment site, such that areas of thinnest skin (i.e. neck and periocular area) are treated with superficial transducers, whereas cheeks and submentum are treated with the deepest transducers, followed by additional treatment with superficial transducers.

Initial treatment protocols suggested a relatively low density of lines placed at just one depth. There has since been a growing trend toward the targeting of multiple depths to affect collagen at multiple treatment planes in order to enhance the efficacy of treatment.[12-14] With dual depth treatment, with the deeper plane treated first, a higher concentration of treatment lines can be delivered in uniform matrices in the targeted location.

Pearl 4

With dual depth treatment, with the deeper plane treated first, a higher cumulative concentration of treatment lines may be delivered in uniform matrices into the targeted anatomy.

Topical skin care products, such as topical retinoids, and alpha- and beta-hydroxy acids, may be discontinued about 2 weeks prior to treatment. All metal facial jewelry is removed prior to treatment. Patients with a history of viral infections can be placed on prophylactic antivirals starting 2 days before and ending 6 days following the procedure. Prior to treatment, the skin is cleaned of any facial products, makeup, lotions or sunscreen. Each treatment region is outlined with a treatment planning card to determine the number of treatment columns. Next, US gel is applied to the target site, and the selected transducer is placed firmly on the skin and activated, with care taken to ensure that the entire transducer is evenly coupled to the skin surface. The US gel may need to be reapplied frequently to ensure proper tissue imaging and coupling, and the acoustic coupling can be visualized and confirmed on the US images. Focal depth can also be visualized and, based on the transducer used and the site targeted, adjustments can be made to align the focal depth with the corresponding tissue layer, from the deep dermis to the SMAS. A parallel linear array of US pulses are then manually delivered with 1 mm to 2 mm spacing between each line. The total number of lines placed in a treatment area depends on the size of the treatment area and particular parameters chosen, with up to 800 lines possible for a full face treatment (Fig. 4.5). Caution should be exercised, and treatment avoided, over soft tissue augmentation material and implants, over the thyroid gland, and inside the orbital rim. Currently, there are no commercially available eye shields that have been shown to effectively block US energy. Following completion of treatment, the US gel is wiped off. Patients may return immediately to their usual activities as there is no downtime associated with this procedure. Medical skincare regimens can be resumed immediately after treatment or within a few days.

Pearl 5

Caution should be exercised (and treatment avoided) over soft tissue augmentation material and implants, over the thyroid gland, and inside the orbital rim.

Although there is a paucity of data regarding the frequency of treatments that patients should receive, it is believed that effective clinical response to US skin tightening lasts approximately 1 year or more depending on

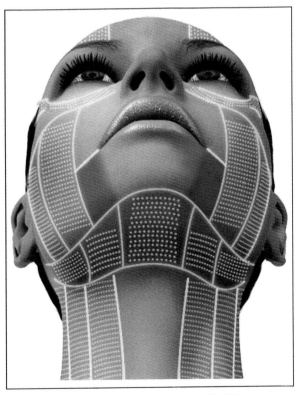

Figure 4.5 Treatment guidelines. Image provided by Ulthera, Inc. with permission.

patients' skin health and underlying rate of aging. Therefore patients can undergo annual maintenance treatments if desired.

Expected outcomes including supporting data from prior studies

Results from several studies have led MFU-V (Ulthera Inc., Mesa, AZ) to receive FDA approval for skin lifting, initially for eyebrow lifting in 2009, followed by an approval for lifting of lax submentum and neck tissue in 2012. Recently, MFU-V has also been used for additional off-label indications. Some examples of MFU-V treated patients are shown in Fig. 4.6.

The first pivotal clinical study in noncadaveric skin was performed by Alam et al.[15] Thirty-five subjects were treated and evaluated for safety and efficacy of treatment. The authors found 86% of the subjects achieved significant improvement 90 days after treatment, as measured by blinded physician assessment. Photographic measurements demonstrated a mean brow lift of 1.7 mm at 90 days. This study led to the first FDA-cleared indication of brow lift for this device.

The second pivotal clinical study was performed by Oni et al.[16] Seventy subjects received MRU-V on the lower face and submentum. All subjects were followed for over 90 days to assess the safety and effectiveness of the treatment. While a total of seven adverse events were reported, only three were considered device/procedure related, and these included urticaria-like linear indurations of the skin within the treated area. All of the events were mild in nature, and resolved completely without sequelae. Quantitative assessment revealed that 72.9% of subjects had a clinical response, defined as a tissue lift of ≥ 20.0 mm^2 of the submental area at 90 days post-treatment. Additionally, 84.3% of subjects who were identified as responders by quantitative assessment were also thus identified in the qualitative masked assessment. In the masked assessment performed by three experienced clinicians, 68.6% of subjects were found to be improved in the submental area and neck. Patient self-report via a satisfaction questionnaire indicated that 67% of subjects noted post-treatment improvement of the face and neck. This study, which demonstrated the safety and effectiveness of MFU-V for submental and neck skin lift, was the basis for the relevant FDA clearance of the device.

Chan et al.[17] evaluated the safety of MFU-V for skin tightening in 49 Chinese subjects. All of the treated subjects underwent full-face and neck treatment with no oral analgesia or topical anesthetics. The authors reported that more than half of the treated subjects rated pain as moderate and experienced only minor, transient adverse effects.

Suh et al.[11] evaluated 22 Korean subjects (Fitzpatrick skin types III–VI) after full-face treatment. All treated subjects reported an improvement, with 91% achieving improvement in numerical score values at the nasolabial fold and jawline. The average improvement was 1.91

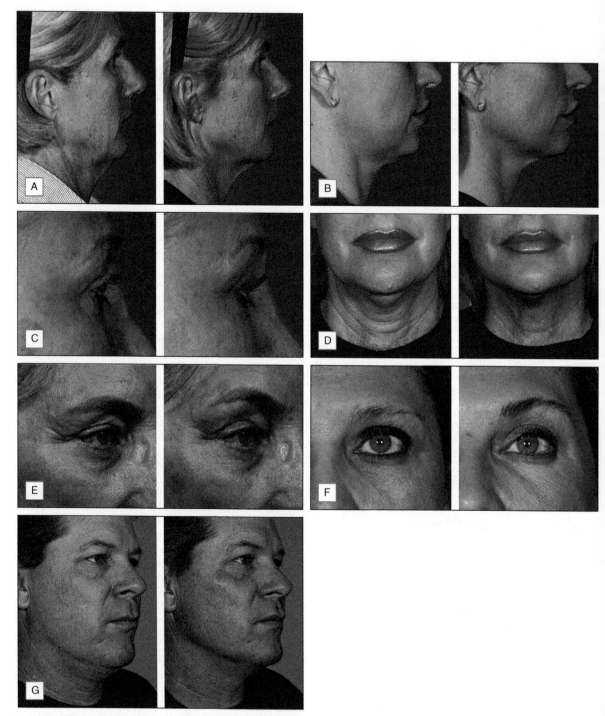

Figure 4.6 MFU-V treated patients. **(A)** Before and 120 days after two treatments. **(B)** Before and 360 days after one treatment. **(C)** Before and 120 days after one treatment. **(D)** Before and 90 days after one treatment. **(E)** Before and 90 days after one treatment. **(F)** Before and 450 days after one treatment. **(G)** Before and 120 days after one treatment.

(scale: 1 = improved, 2 = much improved). Subjectively, 77% of the subjects reported much improvement of nasolabial folds, and 73% reported much improvement of the jawline. The average subjective scores of nasolabial fold and jawline improvement were 1.77 and 1.72, respectively. Skin biopsies obtained from 11 subjects at baseline and 2 months after treatment confirmed an increase in reticular dermal collagen and dermal thickening, with elastic fibers appearing more parallel and straighter than in pre-treatment specimens.

Lee et al.[18] evaluated multipass MFU-V in a study where 10 subjects were treated on the face and neck with the 4 MHz, 4.5 mm probe first, followed by the 7 MHz, 3.0 mm probe. The authors reported an 80% improvement by blinded physician assessment, and 90% reported subjective improvement, 90 days after treatment.

Suh et al.[10] treated 15 subjects with a single pass to the lower infraorbital region with a 7 MHz 3.0 mm transducer and demonstrated objective improvement in all study subjects and subjective improvement in most (86%) of the subjects treated.

Alster and Tanzi first reported the efficacy of MFU-V on body sites.[12] Eighteen study subjects were evaluated using paired areas on the arms, knees, and medial thighs. Dual-plane treatment with the 4 MHz 4.5 mm-depth and 7 MHz 3.0 mm-depth transducers was compared with single-plane treatment with the 4 MHz 4.5 mm-depth transducer alone. Global assessment scores of skin tightening and lifting were determined by two blinded physician raters and graded using a quartile grading scale. At the 6-month follow-up visit, significant improvement was seen in all treated areas, with the upper arms and knees showing more skin lifting and tightening than the thighs. At all three anatomic sites, dual-plane treatment was associated with slightly better clinical scores than single-plane treatment, with this difference potentially secondary to more superficial dermal collagen remodeling in the latter case. Thirteen of the 16 patients were 'highly satisfied' with the procedure and opted to undergo similar micro-focused US treatment of different facial and body areas after the conclusion of the study.

Sasaki and Tevez studied the efficacy of MFU-V for multiple indications.[13] Using the new 10 MHz 1.5 mm superficial transducer, they treated 19 subjects in the periorbital region with 45 lines on each side, and an additional 45 lines using the 7 MHz 3.0 mm transducer at a second depth over the orbital rim. A single treatment produced an average skin elevation between 1 and 2 mm (7–8% increase from baseline) in each of the 19 subjects. Beneficial effects were noted as early as 6 weeks (particularly eyelid and periorbital skin), but the majority of subjects appreciated a smoothing and tightening effect at between 3 and 6 months, when periorbital skin tightening was rated as moderate. Observed responses lasted from about 6 months to 1.5 years. Body sites treated in this study included brachium (44), periumbilicus (6), décolletage (5), knees (4), buttocks (2), inner thighs (1), and hands (1). Treatment protocols varied according to skin

thickness at the treated location. Blinded evaluator assessment scores revealed moderate improvement in the periorbital area, inner brachium, periumbilicus, and knees. Improvement was less consistent on the inner thighs, décolletage, hands, and buttocks, suggesting that further optimization of the treatment process in these areas is needed.

In a larger series of pilot studies and clinical investigations which, in total, included 197 patients, Sasaki and Tevez compared use of horizontal and vertical treatment vectors in the brow and marionette regions while maintaining constant depth and energy.[14] Vertical vectors produced significantly more lifting compared with horizontally placed treatment lines. The authors also showed that significantly greater lifting was achieved at sites with more treatment lines and higher total energy.

A recent study by Fabi and colleagues assessed the efficacy of MFU-V on décolletage laxity and rhytides.[19] The authors reported improvement in rhytides (P<0.0001), with 46% and 62% of subjects showing a 1- to 2-point improvement at days 90 and 180, respectively. Additionally, skin tightening measured as relative to midclavicular to nipple distance (P<0.0001), which decreased from a mean of 20.9 cm (SD 1.57) at baseline to 19.8 cm (SD 1.50) and 19.5 cm (SD 1.59) at days 90 and 180, respectively. Patient satisfaction was high.[18]

Recently reported studies and presentations at scientific meetings have demonstrated a growing number of investigations underway evaluating the applicability of MFU-V for a multitude of treatment sites and indications. Data has been presented supporting the use of MFU-V for wrinkling above the knees,[20] tightening of the neck,[21] and lifting of the buttocks.[22] Additionally, MFU-V is being explored for the treatment of axillary hyperhidrosis[23] and acne. Successful treatment of silicone lip deformity using MFU-V has also been described.[24] The same group has also used MFU-V to control edema and shape the nasal skin after rhinoplasty.[25]

Safety

Overall, MFU-V is associated with an outstanding safety profile, which has led to its widespread adoption and expanding indications. Typical adverse events are mild post-treatment erythema and edema lasting hours to perhaps a day, and resolving spontaneously. Less commonly, purpura may arise, but also soon remits without intervention. Uncommonly, striated linear skin patterns resembling linear wheals or welts may develop at a few focal points; these will recede and disappear within a few weeks but may also be treated with high potency topical corticosteroids for faster resolution. Patients receiving MFU-V do not need to be apprised of impending downtime prior to treatment, and they can continue with normal work and social activities without interruption.

Historically, intraoperative patient discomfort with MFU-V was significant although tolerable, but this issue has been resolved with the advent of new default energy settings on the MFU-V device that have been demonstrated to produce the same size of TCPs. The new settings reduce pain by up to 38% without sacrificing efficacy when the same number of lines are compared in a split face study using old and new settings. Individual published reports of moderate to severe intraoperative pain are therefore based on past experience with older device default settings.[26]

If higher than current default peak fluences are used, sufficient pain management is important to manage the overall treatment experience for the patient. The specific type of pain control varies based on physician preference and the type of treatment performed. MacGregor and Tanzi report using a combination of oral anxiolytics (5–10 mg of diazepam) and intramuscular narcotics (50–75 mg of IM meperidine) 20–30 minutes before treatment to alleviate discomfort in most patients.[27] Other authors have described a variety of methods including use of high dose nonsteroidal anti-inflammatory drugs (NSAIDs), narcotics (oral or intravenous), adjuvant anesthetics (topical or local injection), conscious sedation, distracting massage, and cold techniques.[28] Logically, the higher the energy and the deeper the transducer, the greater is the pain. According to Sasaki and Tevez,[13] the majority of patients who received treatment to the midface and neck did not require a local nerve block or lidocaine whereas patients treated on the forehead/brow occasionally benefitted from local anesthesia or nerve blocks because of the thinness of tissues overlying the frontal bone. Moderate to significant intraoperative pain was experienced most commonly at the décolletage, brachium, knees, and periumbilical sites.[13]

The abovementioned methods of intraoperative pain management are only continuingly clinically relevant for patients and practitioners who choose to use the older default energy settings. The adoption of new treatment paradigms requiring more treatment lines with lower energy per line has largely eliminated the need for active intraoperative pain management orally beyond NSAIDs.

A rare transient complication in the immediate post-treatment period of MFU-V is motor nerve paresis and dysesthesia lasting up to several weeks. Reports are limited to a few individual cases.[27] The areas at the greatest risk for such sequelae are locations where the branches of the facial nerve take a superficial course: the temporal nerve between the lateral canthus and upper helical rim of the ear; the zygomatic nerve as it crosses the zygoma; and the marginal mandibular nerve as it curves over the jaw and onto the anterior neck. Symptoms typically occur within the first 1–12 hours post-treatment and are likely secondary to nerve inflammation. Complete resolution is seen in 2–6 weeks.[27] In patients who notice facial muscle twitching during treatment, icing of the area and possible use of an oral anti-inflammatory medication may be helpful. Sasaki and Tevez reported three patients who developed transient dysesthesia (numbness or hypersensitivity) in a deep branch of the supraorbital nerve, with this lasting for 3–7 days, and four patients who developed numbness along the mandible after treatment on the cheeks, with resolution without sequelae within 2–3 weeks.[14]

Pearl 6

The most concerning complication in the immediate post-treatment period of MFU-V is motor nerve paresis. The areas at greatest risk for injury are locations where the branches of the facial nerve, including the temporal, zygomatic and marginal mandibular nerves, course superficially under the skin. When following the recommended treatment guidelines, these areas are avoided.

Multi-modality procedures

Although there is a lack of published studies with respect to combining US skin tightening with other minimally invasive or noninvasive procedures, it is the experience of these authors that a multi-modality approach is, in fact, effective for the rejuvenation of photoaged skin. For instance, submental fat pads can be removed with liposuction followed by MFU-V skin tightening of the loose overlying skin. In the lower face, MFU-V skin tightening can be followed by soft tissue augmentation to fill residual marionette lines, and perioral and chin depressions. In the periocular area, combination MFU-V treatment and botulinum toxin A injection of the lateral orbicularis oculi muscle can improve both static and dynamic rhytides, while providing a minimal noninvasive brow lift.

CASE STUDY 1

A 47-year-old female presents for a cosmetic consultation. Her medical history is significant for deep venous thrombosis and pulmonary embolism and her only medication is enoxaparin injections daily. The patient's biggest cosmetic concern is excess skin at her chin and upper neck which she reports has become 'looser' over the last decade. She is interested in tightening of the area and has thus decided to seek a cosmetic consultation to address this concern. She has contemplated invasive cosmetic procedures, such as a neck lift or face lift, but has concerns regarding the downtime as well as the potential bleeding risk given her anticoagulation. On physical exam, the patient is noted to have mild laxity of the skin in her neck and jowls. She has never had any surgery in this region and denies any history of filler injections in the area. After a discussion of potential treatment options, including MFU-V skin tightening, she chooses to have an MFU-V skin-tightening treatment. She is counseled that she would likely be able to return to full work and social function immediately, but is made aware of potential bruising if local anesthetic injections are used. She is told that bruising, if it occurs, can usually be concealed with camouflage makeup or appropriate wardrobe choices. The patient proceeds with treatment and presents for follow-up in 3 months. At this follow-up, her jowls and neck appear tighter and she is very pleased with the aesthetic outcome as well as the ease of the procedure.

References

1. Misell L, Li K, Emson CL, et al. Simulation of collagen synthesis in human skin following microfocused ultrasound therapy. Poster session presented at: 12th Annual 2014 South Beach Symposium; 2014 Feb 13-17; Miami Beach, FL.

2. White WM, Makin IR, Barthe PG, et al. Selective transcutaneous delivery of energy to facial subdermal tissues using the ultrasound therapy system [abstr]. Lasers Surg Med 2006;38(Suppl. 18):113.

3. Gliklich RE, White WM, Slayton MH, et al. Clinical pilot study of intense ultrasound therapy to deep dermal facial skin and subcutaneous tissues. Arch Facial Plast Surg 2007;9(2): 88–95.

4. White WM, Makin IR, Barthe PG, et al. Selective creation of thermal injury zones in the superficial musculoaponeurotic system using intense ultrasound therapy: a new target for noninvasive facial rejuvenation. Arch Facial Plast Surg 2007; 9(1):22–9.

5. Laubach HJ, Makin IR, Barthe PG, et al. Intense focused ultrasound: evaluation of a new treatment modality for precise microcoagulation within the skin. Dermatol Surg 2008;34(5): 727–34.

6. White WM, Makin IR, Slayton MH, et al. Selective transcutaneous delivery of energy to porcine soft tissues using intense ultrasound (IUS). Lasers Surg Med 2008;40(2):67–75.

7. Makin IR, Mast TD, Faidi W, et al. Miniaturized ultrasound arrays for interstitial ablation and imaging. Ultrasound Med Biol 2005;31(11):1539–50.

8. Laubach HJ, Barthe PG, Makin IRS, et al. Confined thermal damage with intense ultrasound (IUS) [abstr]. Lasers Surg Med 2006;38(Suppl. 18):32.

9. White WM, Laubach HJ, Makin IRS, et al. Selective transcutaneous delivery of energy to facial subdermal tissues using the ultrasound therapy system [abstract]. Lasers Surg Med 2006;38(Suppl. 18):113.

10. Suh DH, Oh YJ, Lee SJ, et al. A intense-focused ultrasound tightening for the treatment of infraorbital laxity. J Cosmet Laser Ther 2012;14(6):290–5.

11. Suh DH, Shin MK, Lee SJ, et al. Intense focused ultrasound tightening in Asian skin: clinical and pathologic results. Dermatol Surg 2011;37(11):1595–602.

12. Alster TS, Tanzi EL. Noninvasive lifting of arm, thigh, and knee skin with transcutaneous intense focused ultrasound. Dermatol Surg 2012;38(5):754–9.

13. Sasaki GH, Tevez A. Microfocused ultrasound for nonablative skin and subdermal tightening to the periorbitum and body sites. Preliminary report on eighty-two patients. J Cosmet Dermatol Sci Appl 2012;2(2):108–16.

14. Sasaki GH, Tevez A. Clinical efficacy and safety of focused-image ultrasonography: a 2-year experience. Aesthet Surg J 2012;32(5):601–12.

15. Alam M, White LE, Martin N, et al. Ultrasound tightening of facial and neck skin: a rater-blinded prospective cohort study. J Am Acad Dermatol 2010;62(2):262–9.

16. Oni G, Hoxworth R, Teotia S, et al. Evaluation of a microfocused ultrasound system for improving skin laxity and tightening in the lower face. Aesthet Surg J 2014;34(7): 1099–110.

17. Chan NP, Shek SY, Yu CS, et al. Safety study of transcutaneous focused ultrasound for non-invasive skin tightening in Asians. Lasers Surg Med 2011;43(5):366–75.

18. Lee HS, Jang WS, Cha YJ, et al. Multiple pass ultrasound tightening of skin laxity of the lower face and neck. Dermatol Surg 2012;38(1):20–7.

19. Fabi SG, Massaki A, Eimpunth S, et al. Evaluation of microfocused ultrasound with visualization for lifting, tightening, and wrinkle reduction of the decolletage. J Am Acad Dermatol 2013;69(6):965–71.

20. Gold M. A single center, prospective study on the efficacy of the micro-focused ultrasound for the non-invasive treatment of skin wrinkles above the knee. Data Presented at the American Society for Dermatologic Surgery Meeting, Atlanta, GA, 2012.

21. Elm KDL, Schram SE, Wallander ID, et al. Evaluation of a high intensity focused ultrasound system for lifting and tightening of the neck. Data Presented at the American Society for Dermatologic Surgery Meeting, Atlanta, GA, 2012.

22. Goldberg D, Al-Dujaili Z. Micro-focused ultrasound for lifting and tightening skin laxity of the buttock. Data Presented at the American Society for Dermatologic Surgery Meeting, Atlanta, GA, 2012.

23. Nestor MS. Micro-focused ultrasound for the treatment of axillary hyperhidrosis. Data Presented at the American Society for Dermatologic Surgery Meeting, Atlanta, GA, 2012.

24. Kornstein AN. Ulthera for silicone lip correction. Plast Reconstr Surg 2012;129(6):1014e–1015e.

25. Kornstein AN. Ultherapy shrinks nasal skin after rhinoplasty following failure of conservative measures. Plast Reconstr Surg 2013;131(4):664e–666e.

26. Ulthera Update White Paper. Comfort Management. Ulthera, Inc. 3 Feb. 2015 <http://www.ersoyestetik.com/Images/KlinikCalismalar/ULTHERA%20-%20comfort-management-white-paper.pdf>.

27. MacGregor JL, Tanzi EL. Microfocused ultrasound for skin tightening. Semin Cutan Med Surg 2013;32(1):18–25.

28. Brobst RW, Ferguson M, Perkins SW. Ulthera: initial and six month results. Facial Plast Surg Clin North Am 2012;20(2): 163–76, vi.

Subcutaneous Fat: Anatomy, Physiology, and Treatment Indications

5

Misbah Khan, Diana Bolotin, Nazanin Saedi

Key Messages

- Subcutaneous adipose tissue, once considered a passive storage receptacle with a fixed number of cells and limited purpose, is now recognized as a complicated organ with important endocrine and metabolic functions

- Both increased and decreased adipose tissue mass as seen in obesity, anorexia and lipodystrophy, have profound effects on multiple body systems such as the immune, reproductive and hematopoietic systems

- Mature adipocytes exist as two main types: white and brown adipocytes that are distinguished by differences in their color and function and have distinct vascular and nerve supplies

- Treatment options for subcutaneous fat (excess or atrophy) can be broadly categorized as either nonsurgical or surgical

Introduction

Although it is well accepted by dermatologists that subcutaneous fat is an essential component of the skin, the basic science of fat physiology is still a poorly understood 'black hole' in the field of dermatology. Medical disorders related to fat such as panniculitis, lipodystrophies, localized adiposity, and atrophy are commonly treated by dermatologists either by medications or surgical procedures. The demand for procedures that manipulate fat especially for cosmetic enhancement is becoming increasingly popular.[1]

Multiple conditions affect fat distribution in the human body. Studies have shown the association between severe obesity and mortality due to increased rates of cardiovascular disease and diabetes. The type of regional adipose tissue with excess body fat in the upper mid-section of the body called android or male-type obesity represents the entity called visceral obesity. The type of fat distribution associated with accumulation in the lower part of the body or gluteofemoral region is known as gynoid or female type obesity, the excess of which is associated with higher grades of cellulite.

General adiposity (assessed by body mass index [BMI] which is determined by weight/height^2) and abdominal adiposity are associated with a higher risk of death. However, abdominal obesity, which is determined by waist/hip ratio, may be a stronger indicator of obesity than BMI. Visceral and subcutaneous fat have distinct features and excess of either of these may result in a variety of health-related and/or aesthetic concerns.

Subcutaneous fat and gluteofemoral (cellulite) fat

The topographic anatomy of fatty tissue includes two layers that are separated by a superficial fascia. The more external layer or areolar layer consists of vertically oriented globular large adipocytes. The deeper layer, known as the lamellar layer, has horizontally arranged smaller cells with larger and more numerous blood vessels. Women and children tend to have a thicker areolar layer,[2] which, in turn, is thicker in the gluteofemoral regions. Fatty tissue development during puberty is more robust in women than in men. This may be explained by the influence of estrogen as 17β-estradiol stimulates the replication of adipocytes[3] (Fig. 5.1). The adipocytes in the gluteofemoral region are larger and are influenced by female sex hormones These adipocytes are also metabolically more stable and resistant to lipolysis.[4] In addition, estrogen increases the response of the adipocytes to antilipolytic α_2-adrenergic receptors (α_2-ARs).

The only hormones that are able to affect lipolysis in human adipocytes are catecholamines (epinephrine and norepinephrine, which are lipolytic) and insulin (antilipolytic). Functionally, there are marked regional differences in both hormonal responsiveness and metabolic activity of human adipose tissue. Catecholamine-induced lipolytic responsiveness is greater in viscera than in abdominal subcutaneous tissue and gluteofemoral fat cells.[5] The regulation of lipolysis by catecholamines involves AR stimulation of adenylate cyclase via β-ARs (β_1, β_2, and β_3-ARs) and inhibition by α_2-ARs (Fig 5.1). Abdominal and gluteal adipocyte cell size correlates directly with α_2-AR density ($p < 0.1$). The fact that the ratio of α_2-AR to β-AR is higher in the gluteal region than in abdominal adipocytes

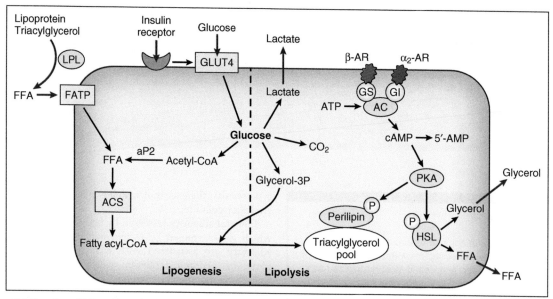

Figure 5.1 Overview of fatty acid uptake, lipogenesis, and lipolysis. Triacylglycerol (TG) hydrolysis leads to lipolysis, whereas fatty acid (FA) uptake and TG synthesis leads to lipogenesis. AC = adenylate cyclase; ACS = acyl-coenzyme A synthase; 5'-AMP = 5'-adenosine monophosphate; ATP = adenosine triphosphate; aP2 = adipocyte binding protein-2; α_2-AR = α_2-adrenoceptor; β-AR = β-adrenoceptor; FATP = fatty acid transport protein; FFA = free fatty acid; GI = inhibitory G protein; GLUT4 = insulin-sensitive glucose transporter; GS = stimulatory G protein; glycerol-3P = glycerol 3-phosphate; HSL = hormone sensitive lipase; LPL = lipoprotein lipase; P = phosphorylation; PKA = protein kinase A *(data modified from Marks DB, Smith CM. Basic medical biochemistry: a clinical approach. Philadelphia: Lippincott Williams & Wilkins; 1996)*

accounts for some of the enhanced responsiveness of abdominal fat cells compared with gluteal fat cells to mixed AR agonists, such as epinephrine and norepinephrine. In addition, abdominal adipocytes have a greater sensitivity to pure β-AR agonists such as isoproterenol. These factors are responsible for enhanced lipolysis of abdominal adipocytes secondary to catecholamine stimulation as compared to gluteal adipose tissue.

Pearl 1

Catecholamine-induced lipolytic responsiveness is greater in visceral fat than in the gluteofemoral or so-called cellulite-prone areas.

Adipose tissue lipoprotein lipase (LPL) directly correlates with the adipose cell size and its affinity for β-AR.[6] Catecholamine-induced lipolysis, as measured by localized LPL release, suggests that abdominal adipocytes have an abundance of β-AR with greater central obesity seen in post-menopausal women as opposed to gynoid feminine type obesity, which is more prevalent in pre-menopausal women. Exogenous estrogen has been shown to have an inconsistent effect on lipolysis. For instance, it was shown to decrease LPL activity in the lower body of pre-menopausal women and yet have the opposite effect in postmenopausal women, again accounting for greater rates of central obesity seen after menopause. Gluteal fat cells are larger in size and richer in α_2-AR in pre-menopausal

and post-menopausal women undergoing hormone replacement therapy.

White and brown adipocytes

Adipocytes are organized in a 'multidepot organ' with only one-third of adipose tissue containing mature adipocytes. The remaining two-thirds consist of a combination of nerves, fibroblasts, and adipocyte precursor cells, or pre-adipocytes (Fig. 5.2). Mature adipocytes exist as two cell types, white adipose tissue (WAT) and brown adipose tissue (BAT), that are distinguished by their color and function. WAT is yellow or ivory and contains predominantly white adipocytes. BAT, which appears brown, contains multilocular brown adipocytes. Compared with WAT, BAT contains a richer vascular tree and denser capillaries in combination with mitochondria, which accounts for its 'brown' color. Both types of adipose tissue are innervated by the noradrenergic sympathetic nervous system.

BAT and WAT are histologically distinct yet interchangeable.[7] Lipids in WAT are organized within one large, 'unilocular' droplet, the size of which exceeds 50 µm. White adipocytes are spherical, allowing for maximum volume expansion within minimal space. The nucleus is compressed to one side because of the high lipid content. Lipids within brown adipocytes are organized into multiple smaller, multilocular droplets. They have higher mitochondrial content packed with cristae within the cytoplasm. Cells are polygonal, have centrally placed

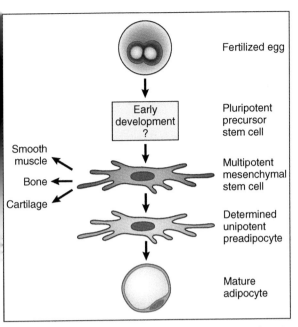

Figure 5.2 Developmental stages of determination and commitment, from egg to mature adipocyte. Diagram represents a model for the development of mature adipocytes from a fertilized egg. Multipotent mesenchymal stem cells can differentiate into cartilage, bone, muscle, and adipocytes *(data from Ntambi J, Kim YC. J Nutr 2000;130(Suppl.): 3122–6 and Gregoire FM, Smas CM, Sul HS. Physiol Rev 1998;78:783–809)*

Pearl 2

Mature adipocytes can be distinguished as either white adipose tissue (WAT) or brown adipose tissue (BAT) with distinct histologic and functional characteristics. Histologically WAT is made up of spherical cells of a wide size range (15–150 µm diameter). The size range is wide due to variation in amount of lipids stored in the lipid vacuole of the adipocyte. Additional cells present within both BAT and WAT include vascular endothelium and neural cells comprising neurovascular bundles supplying it as well as fibroblasts, histiocytes, and mast cells. BAT is made up of smaller 10–25 µm round cells with a cytoplasm rich in mitochondria. Unlike WAT, lipids are stored in small vacuoles within BAT adipocytes and glycogen is abundant. All of these features correspond to the functional differences between the two adipose tissue types. BAT and WAT represent different adipose cell types and have somewhat opposing functions in the body. While WAT acts as an energy storage depot, the main function of BAT is thermogenesis, which involves energy expenditure. Despite these differences in function, it is not unusual to find small islands of BAT within WAT. Furthermore, in states of obesity, BAT can lose its thermogenic function and take on morphological features of WAT.

---

nuclei, and are relatively smaller than WAT, ranging from 20 µm to 40 µm.

WAT is distributed in several anatomically distinct and separate collections or 'depots', namely the subcutaneous and intra-abdominal, each with its own characteristic

metabolic, endocrine, paracrine, and autocrine function[8] (Table 5.1). In humans, BAT is most abundant in newborns and neonates. However in adults, it is also found around many major vessels, in perinephric fat pads and near adrenal glands.[9] In small mammals, such as rodents, BAT persists throughout life. In larger mammals and humans, BAT depots undergo a morphologic transformation in which they rapidly accumulate fat, become unilocular, and lose the ultrastructural and molecular properties that define them, including mitochondria.[10] Because of this, there are very few, if any, collections of BAT in adult humans.

Although WAT and BAT distribution patterns have been well documented, their morphology has been defined on the basis of histologic features alone, which are not sufficient to differentiate between the two. Brown adipocytes may appear white when not stimulated. Likewise, the morphology of white adipocytes changes progressively during fasting. They can become elongated and multilocular, or so-called 'slim'. Because of difficulty differentiating adipocytes based on morphology alone, more advanced techniques are designed to detect the presence of uncoupling protein-1 (UCP-1), a protein that is unique to brown adipocytes. UCP-1 mRNA in adipose tissues is now considered a more accurate method for identifying activated brown adipocytes. Recent polymerase chain reaction (PCR) studies to detect UCP-1 mRNA in adipose tissue from rodents and humans have revealed the existence of scattered BAT within the WAT depots.[11] Furthermore, trans-differentiation of white adipocytes into brown can be induced under certain conditions, thereby refuting the notion that stem cell commitment to, and differentiation into, the white or brown cell lineage is permanent.

WAT and BAT both express many of the same adipocyte-specific genes needed for lipid synthesis and hydrolysis in addition to secreting hormones that regulate energy homeostasis, such as leptin.[12] However, BAT has emerged as an independent organ with specific expression of proteins and unique functions. Mitochondrial protein UCP-1 or thermogenin, which is expressed exclusively in BAT, is responsible for mediating the basic function of brown fat cells – namely, the transfer of energy from nutrition to heat. Being a means of energy expenditure rather than storage, BAT, in theory, may serve a protective function against obesity.[12]

It has been long known that men and women differ in terms of distribution of body fat. Adipose accumulation favors the upper body, trunk and abdomen in men; while women accumulate fat tissue in the lower body, including hips and thighs. This is known as android (male) and gynoid (female) fat distribution patterns. With age, visceral fat accumulation has been shown to increase primarily in men and in menopausal and post-menopausal women. In contrast, pre-menopausal women may accumulate substantial amounts of body fat before starting to accumulate visceral fat. The differences in ways men and women accumulate fat suggest that body fat patterns are strongly influenced by sex hormone homeostasis. The

Table 5.1 Effects of lipid metabolism

Factors	Type of effector	Function
Obesity genes		
Leptin	Endocrine/paracrine	Adipostat signal to brain, decreases food intake, increases energy expenditure, decreases TG synthesis, decreases FA synthesis, increases lipolysis
Agouti	Paracrine	Increases FA synthesis, increases TG synthesis, decreases lipolysis
Cytokines		
TNF-α	Endocrine/paracrine	Proinflammatory effector, decreases pre-adipocyte differentiation, decreases lipogenesis, increases apoptosis, increases lipolysis, increases adipocyte de-differentiation
IL-6	Endocrine/paracrine	Proinflammatory effector, decreases lipogenesis, increases lipolysis
Proteins of lipid metabolism		
GLUT4	Transmembrane glucose protein	+ effector of lipogenesis
LPL	Paracrine	Hydrolyzes lipoprotein-associated Fas, + effector of lipogenesis
Adenosine	Autocrine	Antilipolysis, vasodilator
ALBP/aP2	Intracellular FA binding protein	+ effector of lipolysis
Perilipin	Intracellular lipid droplet associated protein	+ effector of lipolysis
β-AR	Transmembrane catecholamine receptor	+ effector of lipolysis
α_2-AR	Transmembrane catecholamine receptor	(–) effector of lipolysis, antilipolysis
Metabolites		
FFA	Endocrine/paracrine	β-Oxidation, ketone body formation, TG and VLDL synthesis, decreased hepatic and skeletal muscle insulin sensitivity, decreased hepatic insulin clearance, increased gluconeogenesis
Glycerol	Endocrine/paracrine	Increased hepatic TG synthesis

ALBP/aP2, adipocyte-binding lipid protein; α_2-AR, α_2-adrenoceptor; β-AR, β-adrenoceptor; FA, fatty acid; FFA, free fatty acid; GLUT4, insulin dependent glucose transporter; IL-6, interleukin 6; LPL, lipoprotein lipase; TG, triacylglycerol; TNF-α, tumor necrosis factor-α; VLDL, very low density lipoprotein.
Data modified from Wachenberg BL. 2000 Subcutaneous and visceral adipose tissue: their relation to the metabolic syndrome. Endocr Rev 2000;21:697–738.

relationship between estrogens, androgens and abdominal obesity is complex but broadly speaking treatment with testosterone generally leads to a shift to an android pattern of fat distribution. Conversely, estrogen treatment tends to increase fat deposition in all subcutaneous fat depots without increasing visceral fat. While a growing body of data has led to a better understanding of the role of sex hormone homeostasis on adipose tissue distribution and function, more research will be needed to fully understand their physiologic interactions and specific effects on individual adipose compartments.

Treatment indications for subcutaneous fat

The desire to lose weight and to obtain a certain body physique has emerged as an obsession around the world. As a result there has been a tremendous growth in procedures that can reduce stubborn pockets of fat resistant to diet and exercise, both surgically as well as nonsurgically.

The most common reasons for seeking cosmetic removal of fat are related to either obesity itself or the physical stigmata of obesity. Media exposure from television, magazines, and the internet has been shown to correlate obesity with a negative body image and has increased eating disorders.[13] There has been a trend away from the Rubenesque figure to a slender physique, and the continuing presentation of ultra-thin models in the media leads people to internalize the beauty ideal of a lean body. These images in our society make the thin body type the ideal for women and contribute to a high degree of body dissatisfaction. With a focus on a lean body and the limitations of diet and exercise, people seek procedures in order to construct the ideal shape.

The clinical presentation of these concerns is more commonly perceived as localized adiposities alone or in combination with associated skin laxity. The former simply implies the concern of being overweight and its sequelae or perhaps having recently experienced sudden weight loss, while the latter involves the appearance of skin due to underlying adipose tissue anatomy. The pathophysiology of obesity and its treatment, surgical as well as nonsurgical, are vast topics that are beyond the scope of this chapter and will not be discussed herein. However, the various treatment indications for localized adiposities are briefly outlined.

Main body areas to be treated

Localized adiposities can be surgically sculpted from almost any place in the body and face, including, but not limited to, the mandibular border, submental region, breasts, axillae, upper and lower abdomen, flanks, upper and lower back, buttocks, thighs, knees, calves, legs, and ankles. However, nonsurgical body sculpting options are limited in terms of their applications and the predictability of final outcomes. Depending on the device used and the areas treated, one might have to undergo several treatment sessions in order to obtain significant results.

Lipodystrophy

Localized fat adiposities in the face and body can be treated in a variety of ways. Surgical treatment options such as liposuction alone or in combination with laser-assisted lipolysis[14] are the most commonly employed methods. Tumescent liposuction performed under local anesthesia can safely and effectively remove unwanted fat with minimal risk of clinically significant blood loss. Combining laser-assisted lipolysis with Nd:YAG laser therapy can also have an added benefit of skin tightening if desired. However, the improvement in skin laxity is modest at best.

Breast liposuction

Breast reduction by tumescent liposuction or laser-assisted liposuction is a safe and effective procedure for the treatment of breast hypertrophy and related symptoms. Most patients note improvement in symptoms associated with large breasts and the risk of developing worsened nipple ptosis as a result of the procedure has been soundly refuted, although it is true that pre-existing nipple–areola malposition cannot be improved by liposuction alone. Patients undergoing breast liposuction do not appear to develop any significant changes in their mammograms that would obscure detection of malignancy in the future.[15]

Gynecomastia

Gynecomastia can be treated by tumescent liposuction alone and in combination with laser lipolysis. As the male breast is quite fibrous, the heat generated by laser lipolysis facilitates cannula penetration and mobilization of the fat.[16] The cellular disruption (lipolysis), manufactured small tunnels in the breast tissue, and secondary collagen stimulation caused by the procedure all help tissue induce retraction and attenuation of small breast ptosis with concomitant reduction in skin laxity. In the future, there may be a role for noninvasive devices to reduce gynecomastia.

Axillary hyperhydrosis

Tumescent liposuction with curettage is an effective treatment option for patients with hyperhydrosis or osmidrosis refractory to standard medical treatment. Patients with higher sweat rates respond better to this treatment than patients with normal or slightly elevated sweat rates.[17] Liposuction has a higher risk of developing hematoma and erosions if a rasping cannula is used rather than a plain blunt-ended cannula, although it has been suggested that more aggressive curettage with the former is more likely to achieve prolonged remission (Coleman WC, letter in response to Ibrahim O, Kakar R, Bolotin D, Nodzenski M, Disphanurat W, Pace N, Becker L, West DP, Poon E, Veledar E, Alam M). Laser-assisted lipolysis can also be used to cause thermal denaturation of the sweat glands.

Lipomas

Tumescent liposuction has been reported as an alternative to traditional excision for large diffuse lipomas or lipomatosis.[18] The procedure can be safely performed under local anesthesia and in some cases blunt dissection is performed to remove the capsule as well. There is a risk of recurrence and/or incomplete removal can occur with this procedure if the entire lipoma is tightly pseudoencapsulated and eludes complete fracture and mobilization. However, tumescent liposuction may be the preferred option if the risk of scarring associated with open excision is of concern.

Conclusion

Adipose tissue has a complex interaction with the endocrine and circulatory systems. Distribution of body adipose depots varies between men and women and changes during the aging process. As mentioned, men and women have different distributions of body fat. Men have an android fat distribution pattern with adipose accumulation favoring the upper body, trunk and abdomen. Women have a gynoid fat distribution pattern with adipose accumulating in the lower body including hips and thighs. With age, visceral fat accumulation has been shown to increase primarily in men and in menopausal and post-menopausal women. Visceral obesity is associated with increased cardiovascular risk. Increase in visceral obesity appears to be controlled by a critical balance of sex hormones as well as individual hormonal responsiveness of the fat tissue. Thus, future studies of homeostasis of subcutaneous fat tissue may shed light on its interaction with visceral fat distribution. Both superficial and deep layers of subcutaneous fat are related to the skin surface alterations that characterize cellulite and localized adiposities, which play an important role in each individual's physical appearance. With the sociocultural influences that focus on a slim physique, there has been a rising demand for body contouring. Both surgical and noninvasive treatments for fat reduction have become increasingly popular.

References

1. Matarasso A, Kim RW, Kral JG. The impact of liposuction on body fat. Plast Reconstr Surg 1998;102:1686–9.
2. Rossi AB, Vergnanini AL. Cellulite: a review. J Eur Acad Dermatol Venerol 2000;14:251–62.
3. Krotkiewski M, Bjorntorp P, Sjostrom L, Smith U. Impact of obesity on metabolism in men and women. Importance of regional tissue distribution. J Clin Invest 1983;72:1150–62.
4. Khan MH, Victor F, Rao BK, Sadick NS. Treatment of cellulite. Part 1. Pathophysiology. J Am Acad Dermatol 2010;62:361–70.
5. Wahrenberg H, Lonnqvist F, Arner P. Mechanisms underlying regional differences in lipolysis in human adipose tissue. J Clin Invest 1989;84:458–67.
6. Berman DM, Nicklas BJ, Rogus EM, et al. Regional differences in adrenoreceptor binding and fat cell lipolysis in obese, postmenopausal women. Metabolism 1998;47:467–73.
7. Cinti S. Adipocyte differentiation and transdifferentiation: plasticity of adipose organ. J Endocrinol Invest 2002;25:823–35.
8. Smith SR, Lovejoy JC, Greenway F, et al. Contributions of total body abdominal fat, subcutaneous adipose tissue to the metabolic complications of obesity. Metabolism 2001;50:425–35.
9. Houstek J, Vizek K, Pavelka S, et al. Type II iodothyronine 5′-deiodinase and uncoupling protein in brown adipose tissue of human newborns. J Clin Endocrinol Metabol 1993;77(2):382–7.
10. Himms-Hagen J. Does brown adipose tissue have a role in the physiology or treatment of human obesity? Rev Endocrinol Metabol Disord 2001;2:395–401.
11. Penicaud L, Cousin B, Leloup C, et al. The autonomic nervous system, adipose tissue plasticity and energy balance. Nutrition 2000;16:903–8.
12. Avram AS, Avram MM, James WD. Subcutaneous fat in normal and diseased states: 2 Anatomy and physiology of white and brown adipose tissue. J Am Acad Dermatol 2005;53:671–83.
13. Derenne JL, Beresin EV. Body image, media, and eating disorders. Acad Psychiatry 2006;30:257–61.
14. Kim KH, Geronemus RG. Laser lipolysis using a novel 1064-nm Nd:YAG laser. Dermatol Surg 2006;32:241–8.
15. Mellul SD, Dryden RM, Remigio DJ, Wulc AE. Breast reduction performed by liposuction. Dermatol Surg 2006;32:112–33.
16. Ichikawa K, Miyasaka M, Tanaka R, et al. Histologic evaluation of pulsed Nd:YAG laser for laser lipolysis. Lasers Surg Med 2005;36:43–6.
17. Tsai RY, Lin JY. Experience of tumescent liposuction in the treatment of osmidrosis. Derm Surg 2001;27:446–8.
18. Choi CW, Kim J, Moon SE, et al. Treatment of lipomas assisted with tumescent liposuction. J Eur Acad Dermatol Venerol 2007;21:243–6.

Cryolipolysis: Fat Reduction

Roberta Spencer Del Campo, Jeffrey Orringer

6

Key Messages

- Cryolipolysis is a novel approach to noninvasive subcutaneous fat reduction
- It is both safe and effective with essentially no post-procedure downtime
- Commonly treated areas include flanks, upper and lower abdomen, and back fat pads
- The pre-procedure consultation is critical to selecting appropriate patients for this treatment
- Erythema, mild edema and petechiae are common immediate sequelae that typically resolve within a week
- A transient reduction in sensation (i.e. paresthesia) may also be experienced but this typically resolves within a few weeks
- No significant negative long-term sequelae have been observed to date

Introduction

As body contouring and selective fat removal have become a frequent goal of aesthetically-oriented procedures, there have been numerous efforts to develop a technique that is effective yet noninvasive and leads to minimal or no patient downtime. For decades, liposuction has been a gold standard procedure in fat removal. Although this treatment is highly effective for high volume localized fat removal, it requires small incisions in the skin followed by various modalities to loosen the adipose tissue prior to suctioning excess fat through a cannula. Due to the moderately invasive nature of liposuction, it can uncommonly lead to complications including hematomas, infection, scarring, sensation changes, nonuniform fat reduction, and damage to underlying structures. Because of the potential side effects and social downtime associated with liposuction and surgical approaches to fat reduction, there have been recent and ongoing efforts to develop truly noninvasive techniques to selectively decrease adipose tissue. Evolving methods developed to date include ultrasound, radiofrequency, infrared light and laser treatments, all of which have been associated with variable results and sometimes limited efficacy. A recent alternative approach has been founded on the concept of selective cryolipolysis. Cryolipolysis literally means 'freezing of fat' and this treatment modality utilizes targeted cold exposure to produce selective fat reduction without damaging overlying skin or surrounding tissue. As this treatment is completely noninvasive, there is no post-procedure downtime and little risk for significant long-term side effects or complications.

Pathophysiology/mechanism of action

Initial hints that fat cells are preferentially sensitive to cold exposure included two clinical entities – the well-known 'popsicle panniculitis' and the so-called 'equestrian panniculitis'. Popsicle panniculitis was initially described as early as the 1960s when it was noted that children who sucked on frozen treats for extended periods of time developed inflammation and subsequent loss of buccal fat tissue.[1,2] Similar findings of inflammation and fat loss were later noted in female equestrian riders who wore tight pants in cold climates. This latter clinical scenario was therefore termed 'equestrian panniculitis'.[3] Together, these findings ultimately provoked various animal and clinical studies designed to explore the link between cold exposure and selective fat destruction.

The initial animal studies were performed by Manstein and colleagues and consisted of three complementary experiments involving Yucatan pigs.[4] The first of the series was considered an exploratory study designed to determine the feasibility of noninvasive, cold induced, selective destruction of subcutaneous fat. In this initial project, a black Yucatan pig was subjected to a slightly convex circular copper plate that was pressed firmly against the skin surface and was cooled by antifreeze solution set at −7 °C. The cold exposure time varied between 5 and 21 minutes and was repeated at several different locations. Following cold exposure, the pig was monitored for 3.5 months and researchers observed the appearance and persistence of localized fat loss. During this time, it was noted that the pig developed focal indentations at the sites of contact with the cooling device. As compared with adjacent untreated areas, histologic sections of the treated sites demonstrated an estimated 80% loss of the superficial layer of adipose tissue for a total loss of 40% of the measured thickness of the subcutaneous tissue. There was also a marked reduction in the distance between fat septa with no evidence of surrounding skin injury and only transient hyperpigmentation in the overlying skin.

In a subsequent dosimetry study, four pigs were treated with a prototype device (Zeltiq Aesthetics Inc., Pleasanton, CA) containing a thermoelectric cooling element. The animals studied were treated with either a flat device applicator pressed firmly against the skin or with the treated skin folds captured between two cooling plates. The cooling plates were kept at a pre-set temperature ranging from −1 °C to −7 °C for 10 minutes. Animals were sacrificed at selected time points ranging from immediately to 28 days post-procedure. Test sites and surrounding areas were assessed clinically, with an ultrasound device, and with histologic sections. Findings included clinically obvious indentations at various test sites where the cooling plate applicator was used. However, there was no apparent clinical change at locations where the flat applicator was used. Using an ultrasound device, treated areas were assessed at 30 days post-treatment and an approximately 3 mm thickness of fat loss was demonstrated as compared with surrounding untreated skin. Furthermore and perhaps most importantly, the histologic findings supported the theory that cold exposure may induce selective fat loss without damage to surrounding tissues. As seen in Table 6.1, histologic sections immediately following the procedure demonstrated normally shaped adipocytes and no inflammatory cells. By day 2 after cold exposure, adipocytes again appeared normal, but there was evidence of localized inflammation in the subcutaneous tissue. Specifically, the inflammation consisted of clusters of neutrophils and monocytes in a lobular pattern. By day 14 following treatment, there was

evidence of a reduction in adipocyte size as well as a heavier inflammatory infiltrate consisting of occasional macrophages. And finally, by day 30, there was an even greater reduction in adipocyte size and an increased density of macrophages, suggesting more significant phagocytosis of the damaged adipocytes. Importantly, blinded grading of the degree of inflammation suggested relatively greater adipocyte damage and a heavier inflammatory infiltrate at lower temperatures.

> **Pearl 1**
>
> Selective cooling of superficial fat leads to apoptosis of adipocytes followed by gradual clearing of the apoptotic debris by inflammatory cells. As this is a selective process, the overlying epidermis and dermis are generally unaffected and surrounding, untreated skin is left uninjured.

Although the exact mechanism(s) of action remain somewhat unclear, the pre-clinical studies noted above confirmed the phenomenon of selective cryolipolysis with regulated cold exposure leading to apoptosis of adipocytes. These findings ultimately led to the development of the Zeltiq system (Zeltiq, Pleasanton, CA) which is the first device developed for human use. This system consists of a control unit with a cup-shaped applicator that uses vacuum suction to position the excess adipose tissue between two cooling plates. The cooling of the plates is modulated by a thermoelectric cooling element which extracts energy from the underlying adipose tissue without damaging the overlying skin. The temperature is controlled and kept constant by sensors embedded in the cooling plate. Further, the device's applicators are designed to apply sufficient pressure to nearly eliminate cutaneous blood flow in the treated skin, eliminating convective heat exchange. Together the cooling applicator and its 'folded' design result in selective cooling of fat while extracting energy and ultimately causing apoptosis of adipocytes. This is followed by a gradual inflammatory response leading to even more adipocyte damage and eventual phagocytosis of the apoptotic debris.

Patient selection

Appropriate patient selection is vital to ensure positive results and patient satisfaction. Ideal candidates for cryolipolysis are those individuals who are relatively fit with stubborn areas of fat accumulation that do not respond to diet and exercise. Ideal areas to treat include the flanks, abdomen, and mid to lower back. Other common areas where fat may accumulate, such as the hips, thighs, buttocks, upper arms, and neck, may also respond well to this procedure and, therefore, further investigation of additional potential treatment sites is both warranted and ongoing. The 'sandwich' design of cryolipolysis treatment heads has been modified to provide separate attachments appropriate for treatment of various body sites and sizes

Table 6.1 Histologic changes over 30 days post-treatment

Day post-treatment	Histological findings
Day 0	Within first hour, normally shaped and sized adipocytes with no inflammatory cells
Day 2	Clusters of inflammatory cells (mainly neutrophils) surrounding individual adipocytes
Day 14	Dense lymphocytic infiltrate with occasional macrophages and some reduction of adipocyte size
Day 30	Dense lymphocytic infiltrate, multinucleated giant cells (macrophages), further reduction of adipocyte size

Adapted from Manstein D, Laubach H, Watanabe K, et al. Selective cryolysis: a novel method for noninvasive fat removal. Lasers Surg Med 2008;40(9):595–604.

of local adiposities. Importantly, as cryolipolysis does not directly affect the epidermis, patients of all Fitzpatrick skin types and ethnicities may be safely treated.

Pearl 2

Ideal candidates for cryolipolysis include fit individuals who want to treat localized fat bulges that are unresponsive to diet and exercise without surgical intervention and, therefore, no associated downtime.

In comparison to traditional surgical treatments for excess adipose tissue, cryolipolysis may be performed as an outpatient procedure in a clinic setting. There is no need for sterile conditions, anesthesia, or incisions and these factors both allow the procedure to be done at a comparatively lower cost and eliminate most of the potential risks associated with surgical procedures. Therefore, patients who wish to minimize cost and avoid an invasive procedure requiring anesthesia, significant surgical risks, and post-treatment downtime are also ideal candidates.

Patients who wish to undergo a noninvasive procedure with little associated discomfort or pain may also benefit from this treatment. A recent European study focusing on safety, tolerance, and patient satisfaction reported that 96% of 518 patients treated noted minimal to tolerable pain levels associated with the cryolipolysis procedure. Pain that was reported as 'severe' was only noted in 4% of patients and only occurred during the initial 5 minutes of treatment.[5] In general, patients are uncomfortable for the first few minutes of each 1-hour treatment; after this initial period of feeling very cold at the site of treatment, sensation diminishes and the remainder of the treatment is typically minimally uncomfortable.

It should also be noted that, on average, this procedure only reduces excess adipose tissue in a given area by approximately 20–25% per treatment and may take up to 12–16 weeks for maximal improvement.[6] Typically, 1–3 treatments are performed at a given site to induce modest reduction of a medium-sized local adiposity. Therefore, in general, cryolipolysis is not a replacement for the maximal fat reduction possible through more invasive procedures, such as liposuction or a surgical 'tummy tuck,' and it is not ideal for a patient looking for immediate improvement. Cryolipolysis has no utility in the treatment of visceral adipose tissue (which does not respond) or as a weight loss tool, and it has not been shown to impact insulin resistance.

In summary, the common candidate for cryolipolysis is willing to expect a more modest, gradual change in appearance than one would achieve with surgical treatments or liposuction, has a well-defined superficial layer of diet- and exercise-resistant adipose tissue at the abdomen, flanks, or back, and wishes to avoid the risks and recovery period associated with relatively more invasive fat reduction procedures.

CASE STUDY 1
'On further exam'

A 60-year-old male presents for consultation. He is 5'10" and 220 pounds and is interested in cryolipolysis for his mid section. On examination, you note a protuberant abdomen, which is firm to palpation. Pinch test is negative. Per your exam, you determine that his excess abdominal adipose tissue is primarily visceral in nature and, therefore, would not be responsive to this treatment. You continue your exam noting additional excess adipose tissue along his flanks. Pinch test is positive. You inform the patient that although his abdominal adipose tissue is visceral in nature and would not respond well to cryolipolysis, his flanks would be ideal for this procedure. One week later he returns to your office for treatment of his flanks.

Typical treatment course

Patients should be instructed to arrive at least 30 minutes prior to their scheduled treatment time. This will ensure enough time to take carefully standardized pre-treatment photographs and to obtain a pre-treatment weight. It is the authors' opinion that pre-treatment circumferential measurements are not particularly helpful as it is difficult to standardize these measurements and thus eventual comparisons with follow-up measurements may not be accurate.

Standardization of photographs will allow for a more accurate comparison of pre- and post-treatment images. Some suggestions include selecting a designated area where a solid color background, such as a blue or black sheet, can be hung. A pre-set distance from this background should be determined and the floor should be marked with a piece of duct tape. This location will signify where the camera will be positioned, ensuring a consistent distance from patient to camera. The camera should also be at a consistent height. This can be achieved using a camera tripod, locked at a pre-selected height. The pre-selected distance and height measurements for the photographs should be added to the patient's medical record. In addition, the manufacturer provides a 'wheel' to be placed on the floor on which patients stand during photographs. This enhances the uniformity of patient positioning and camera angles. Furthermore, when photographs are taken, patients should wear loose fitting clothing so as to not alter the appearance of their excess adipose tissue; for example, large loose fitting shorts may be obtained from the manufacturer and should be worn during both pre- and post-treatment photographs.

After the steps outlined above are completed, the areas to be treated are marked with a pen to ensure proper positioning of the vacuum applicator. It is important to not only mark the apex of the excess adipose tissue but to also mark the borders of where the applicator will be placed. Cardboard cutouts mimicking the shapes of the various vacuum applicators may be obtained from the

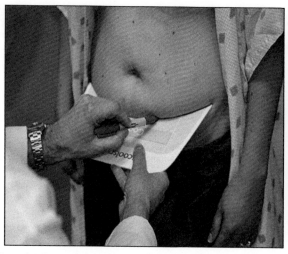

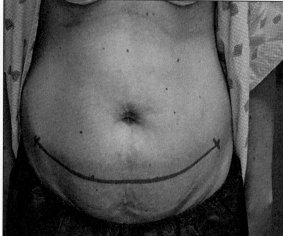

Figure 6.1 Appropriate marking of the area to be treated

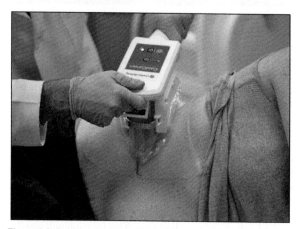

Figure 6.2 Applicator placement on patient

manufacturer and are extremely useful in assisting with pre-procedure planning and patient marking. An example can be seen in Figure 6.1.

After the patient is marked for applicator placement, the patient is positioned on the examination table or a comfortable chair. Commonly, the patient's back is kept at a slight incline to allow for an easier grasp of the excess adipose tissue during vacuum applicator placement. To protect the overlying skin, a gel pad is placed over the pre-marked area. It is important that the gel pad covers all skin that will come in contact with the vacuum device – particularly skin located in the center of the treatment area that will be pulled between the applicator's cooling plates. The applicator is then positioned over the marked area and the handpiece is turned on, creating a vacuum, which draws the excess adipose tissue in between the cooling plates (Fig. 6.2). The clamping effect of the plates not only allows for more direct contact of the cooling plates to the adipose tissue, it also locally restricts blood-flow, allowing for more effective cooling. Prior to activat-

ing the device's cooling mechanism, it is important to ensure there is good vacuum suction with adequate excess adipose tissue drawn between the cooling plates. It is also important to ensure that the handpiece is placed within the pre-marked borders. Patient comfort is also assessed and patient positioning is addressed before activating the cooling cycle because excessive movement may cause the applicator to 'pop off' during treatment. The authors have found it helpful to place pillows around the applicator to help maintain appropriate positioning and adequate contact throughout the procedure. It is also useful to ensure that the gel pad is in place between the skin's surface and the cooling plates circumferentially around the applicator.

Once tissue capture, patient comfort, and gel pad placement are confirmed, the cooling plates are turned on and the treatment cycle begins. The standard cycle is 60 minutes per treatment area. During this time, patients are free to read or rest. They are left with a nurse call-button and their comfort may be assessed as appropriate during the treatment. On completion of the cycle, the applicator is removed, revealing treated tissue that is firm, cool, erythematous, raised above the normal tissue plane, and molded to the shape of the applicator (Fig. 6.3A). Some compare this appearance to the shape of a cold stick of butter. It is believed that post-treatment firm massage of the treatment area for approximately 5 minutes improves disadhesion and mechanical rupture of the crystalized adipocytes with possibly improved clinical results (Fig. 6.3B, C).[6]

Pearl 3

Standardizing photographs by maintaining a consistent background, camera set-up and patient positioning will help to ensure an accurate comparison of before and after treatment photographs.

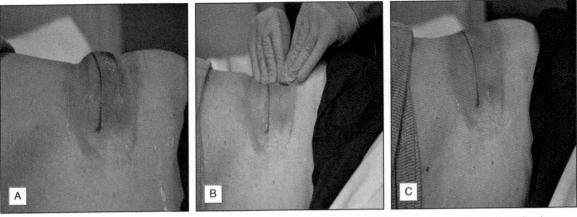

Figure 6.3 (A) Immediately post-treatment. This has been compared to a 'stick of butter'. **(B)** Massaging the area for 5 minutes breaks up crystal formation. **(C)** Appearance of treated area post-massage

Expected outcomes

As mentioned previously, several studies to date have demonstrated a measurable reduction in superficial subcutaneous tissue after contact with a cooling device. The initial animal studies, on Yucatan pigs, performed by Manstein and colleagues demonstrated clinical indentations at sites of skin contact with a prototype cooling device.[4] The indented sites were compared with adjacent, untreated areas. Pigs are known to have two distinct layers within their subcutaneous tissue and gross and histologic sections of the treated sites demonstrated an estimated 80% reduction in the thickness of the superficial fat layer and a total reduction of 40% of the thickness of the overall adipose tissue in the area. A follow-up clinical study by Dover and colleagues in which 32 patients were treated with cryolipolysis to their flanks and back fat pads demonstrated an average reduction in subcutaneous tissue of 22.4% at 4 months follow-up.[7,8] In a separate study consisting of 10 treated patients, nine of whom were assessed, there was a 25.5% reduction in the thickness of the adipose layer at 6 months post-treatment.[9] Furthermore, although long-term studies are lacking, a recent case study of two male subjects demonstrated durable clinical reductions in treated areas at 2 and 5 years post-treatment.[10]

Based on these studies it has been the authors' practice to educate patients during their consultation visit that there will be, on average, an approximate reduction of 20–25% in the thickness of the excess adipose tissue per treatment. Therefore, if a greater reduction is desired, additional treatments to the same area may be planned. Additionally, as noted previously, the post-procedure fat reduction seen after cryolipolysis is a gradual process and it may take 12–16 weeks to achieve the maximal clinical benefit of a given treatment session (Figs 6.4 and 6.5).

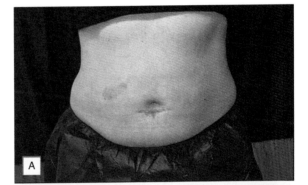

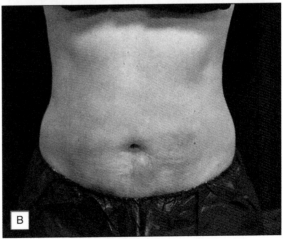

Figure 6.4 (A) Pre-treatment. **(B)** 12 weeks post-treatment to upper and lower abdomen using cryolipolysis

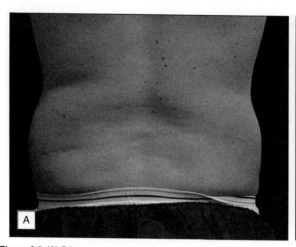 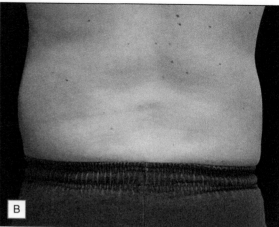

Figure 6.5 (A) Prior to treatment of bilateral flanks. **(B)** 6 weeks post-treatment with cryolipolysis

Pearl 4

On average, patients can expect a 20–25% reduction in the thickness of the treated subcutaneous layer per treatment. It may take 12–16 weeks for maximal clinical improvement before an additional treatment, if appropriate, is undertaken.

CASE STUDY 2
'It takes time'

A female in her 30s presents for cryolipolysis of her flanks. You treat bilaterally and recommend follow-up in 2–3 months to evaluate her progress. She contacts your clinic 3 weeks later, worried that she has only seen slight improvement. You remind her that it may take up to 16 weeks to see the final results of a treatment session. She expresses her understanding and returns for her follow-up appointment 14 weeks post-procedure. At her appointment, she is extremely happy that her pants fit better and she has noticed a significant improvement in the appearance of her 'love handles'. You obtain a second set of photographs and compare them with her pre-treatment images. On comparison, there is clear improvement in the patient's appearance with a clinically obvious localized decrease in excess adipose tissue of the flanks despite the fact that the patient's weight has remained stable.

Safety

Cryolipolysis utilizing a proprietary technique called CoolSculpting® (Zeltiq) is considered a safe, noninvasive, FDA-approved treatment for localized truncal fat reduction. As compared with liposuction or other surgical treatments, cryolipolysis is entirely noninvasive and does not require anesthesia. There is little concern for the develop-ment of infection, hematomas, or scarring with this procedure.

Not uncommonly, erythema, swelling, petechiae or larger bruises, tenderness, and transient decreased sensation may occur. Most of these relatively minor localized side effects typically resolve within 1 week of treatment. A recent study noted a somewhat longer mean duration of sensory nerve changes (mean of 3.6 weeks) with patients generally noting a partial decrease in sensation at the treatment sites. Importantly, in this study, histologic stains demonstrated no significant long-term changes in nerve fiber structure and no long-term sensation loss was noted.[9] In comparison, transient increased sensitivity has also been noted in a relatively small number of patients. One study reported an incidence of 2.5% within the first few days of treatment.[5] Some patients may also report an intermittent cramping sensation or even sharp, localized pain that may be particularly notable at night. Importantly, these sensory changes are generally not severe enough to affect normal daily activities and typically resolve within 3–4 weeks.

In addition to possible alterations in sensation, there was also initial concern that cryolipolysis may theoretically increase blood lipid levels secondary to fat mobilization. Studies to date have not supported this concern. One notable study by Zelickson et al. included three Yucatan pigs and one Yorkshire pig that were treated with a prototype cooling device at temperatures ranging from –5 °C to –8 °C for 10 minutes.[11] Blood samples were then obtained at 1 hour, 1 day, 1 week, and monthly for 3 months post-treatment. These values were compared to an initial sample taken prior to treatment after a 12-hour fast. Other than a temporary decrease in serum triglycerides immediately following the procedure (attributed to fasting prior to and during general anesthesia), the authors reported no significant changes in lipid levels following the cold exposure.[11] A later study involving 40 human subjects, performed by Klein and colleagues in 2009, also showed no significant increases in serum lipid levels or liver function tests. The lack of elevated lipid levels is thought to be due to the gradual release of fat following adipocyte apoptosis over several weeks post-treatment.[12]

In the authors' clinical practice a detailed consent form is signed by all patients prior to the procedure. In addition to the more common, minor side effects noted above, our consent also notes the possibility of more rare side effects, including: a partial or complete lack of response; post-treatment contour defects; skin dyspigmentation; firmness of treated areas; enlargement of the treated areas; or the formation of discrete nodules post-procedure. According to a recent study, 2.5% of patients reported nodules or diffuse infiltration in the treatment area.[5] This was associated with tenderness and erythema that was improved with ibuprofen or acetaminophen. All cases resolved spontaneously within 1–3 weeks. Interestingly, this study noted greater efficacy when infiltration was noted, suggesting that a greater inflammatory response triggers a more pronounced treatment response.[5]

Pearl 5

Cryolipolysis has not been shown to increase serum lipid levels or negatively alter liver function tests. Furthermore, there have been no reported long-term sensory alterations or damage to adjacent skin tissue reported with this treatment.

References

1. Rotman H. Cold panniculitis in children. Arch Dermatol 1966;94:720–1.
2. Epsein EH Jr, Oren ME. Popsicle panniculitis. N Engl J Med 1970;282(17):966–7.
3. Beacham BE, Cooper PH, Buchanan CS, Weary PE. Equestrian cold panniculitis in women. Arch Dermatol 1980;116(9):1025–7.
4. Manstein D, Laubach H, Watanabe K, et al. Selective cryolysis: a novel method for non-invasive fat removal. Lasers Surg Med 2008;40(9):595–604.
5. Dierickx CC, Mazer JM, Sand M, et al. Safety, tolerability, and patient satisfaction with noninvasive cryolipolysis. Dermatol Surg 2013;39(8):1209–16.
6. Jalian HR, Avram HM. Cryolipolysis: a historical perspective and current clinical practice. Semin Cutan Med Surg 2013;32(1):31–4.
7. Dover J, Burns J, Coleman S, et al. A prospective clinical study of non-invasive cryolipolysis for subcutaneous fat layer reduction. Interim report of available subject data. Lasers Surg Med 2009;S21:45.
8. Avram MM, Harry RS. Cryolipolysis for subcutaneous fat layer reduction. Lasers Surg Med 2009;41:703–8.
9. Coleman SR, Sachdeva K, Egbert BM, et al. Clinical efficacy of non-invasive cryolipolysis and its effects on peripheral nerves. Aesthetic Plast Surg 2009;33:482–8.
10. Bernstein EF. Longitudinal evaluation of cryolipolysis efficacy: two case studies. J Cosmet Dermatol 2013;12(2):149–52.
11. Zelickson B, Egbert BM, Preciado J, et al. Cryolipolysis for noninvasive fat cell destruction: initial results from a pig model. Dermatol Surg 2009;35(10):1462–70.
12. Klein KB, Zelickson B, Riopelle JG, et al. Non-invasive cryolipolysis for subcutaneous fat reduction does not affect serum lipid levels or liver function tests. Lasers Surg Med 2009;41(10):785–90.

Radiofrequency Treatment: Fat Reduction

7

Laurel Morton, Robert A. Weiss

Key Messages

- Radiofrequency (RF) devices are a recent advancement in noninvasive technology designed to reduce the appearance of fat. Often, they are based on the emission of an electromagnetic field that results in a current running through subcutaneous tissue and causing bulk heating. These innovations are safe with low side effect profiles, and they can be used on all skin types

- Ideal patients for most of these procedures are healthy with relatively discrete sites of unwanted fat such as those at the abdomen, 'love handles', and thighs. There is no downtime associated with these procedures and they are an alternative to surgical interventions for body contouring

- There are multiple variations of the RF technology designed to target subcutaneous tissue. They include, but are not limited to, tripolar and unipolar devices as well as those which are based on the emission of nonionizing radiation

- Data remains in its early stages and is limited. However, RF devices targeting subcutaneous tissue are reported to reduce circumference of the abdomen and thighs and in some cases show a decreased thickness in subcutaneous tissue via ultrasound and histopathologic data

Introduction

A decade ago, the only reliable methods by which to reduce fat and its appearance were invasive and included procedures such as abdominoplasty and liposuction. These surgical techniques posed issues of significant downtime and potential side effects related to the procedures themselves and any necessary general anesthesia. Fortunately, within the last decade, multiple noninvasive technologies have been developed to visibly decrease the appearance of fat and, in some cases, show a histologic decrease in subcutaneous volume and a diminution of adipocyte size and integrity. Radiofrequency (RF) is a particularly interesting modality for fat reduction.

Pearl 1

Ideal patients for radiofrequency-induced fat reduction are healthy with a normal BMI and discrete areas of unwanted fat such as those located at the abdomen, waist and thighs.

When speaking of cosmetic interventions, the first RF device was Federal Drug Administration (FDA)-approved for wrinkle reduction in 2002 (ThermaCool®, Thermage®, Haywood, CA).[1] Currently, RF is applied to a much broader range of treatments including skin rejuvenation, tightening and wrinkle reduction, acne and acne scarring, improved appearance of cellulite, and fat reduction. Its wide array of applications can be explained by a multitude of unique and specific RF technologies that have been developed, several of which are applied for fat reduction.

Radiofrequency refers to radiation at the far end of the electromagnetic spectrum, which has a frequency between 3 kHz and 300 MHz (Fig. 7.1).[1] Energy emitted at these frequencies is not strong enough to be ionizing.[2] Unlike laser devices, which emit energy in the form of a unique wavelength of light, RF devices emit energy in the form of electromagnetic waves that induce an alternating current in the targeted tissue. Tissue is composed of individual molecules, which are electrical dipoles. When current or electrons flow through a material, the dipoles align with the current and then change orientation millions of times per second as the current alternates. Each tissue type has a unique resistance to this movement of molecules, otherwise known as impedance. The movement of dipoles against resistance can be thought of as a type of friction that leads to energy in the form of heat, thereby converting electrical energy into thermal energy. By Ohm's law, energy emitted by an RF device is proportional to the current it produces (I), the specific impedance of a particular tissue (Z) and time (t):[2,3]

$$\text{Energy (joules)} = I^2 \times Z \times t$$

Importantly, RF devices have some advantages over lasers that allow them to target subcutaneous tissue. Electromagnetic waves lose energy exponentially as they travel across tissue. High frequencies and small wavelengths

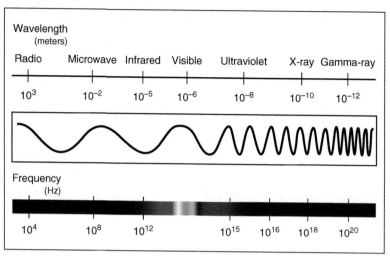

Figure 7.1 The electromagnetic spectrum

used by laser light attenuate quickly, while RF energy does not and is therefore able to penetrate deeper fatty tissue.[4] RF is not dissipated by scatter or absorbed by epidermal melanin, and, unlike some forms of laser energy,[2] all skin types may be treated with RF. The effect of laser energy is described by the concept of selective photothermolysis and is relatively pinpointed. Conversely, the fact that RF energy is not localized is important for causing bulk heating,[4] which is a quality necessary to reach adequate treatment temperatures in larger areas. When correct frequencies are chosen, subcutaneous tissue may be particularly targeted for heating.[5,6]

Technology and mechanism of action

Crucially, RF results in heating when applied to tissue. In ex vivo analysis, when adipocytes are heated, their viability decreases. To illustrate this, Franco and colleagues demonstrated that 3 days after cultured adipocytes are heated to 45 °C and 50 °C, there is only 89% and 20% viability of cells, respectively. Cells heated to 45 °C for 3 minutes show only 40% viability.[5] At least one group has demonstrated that heating secondary to RF causes cell-mediated death or apoptosis.[6] RF technology makes use of this adipocyte instability in order to reduce its appearance and/or volume.

Historically speaking, RF devices were either monopolar or bipolar. Monopolar describes a system in which the electric current is dispelled by a handpiece into the skin and exits the body through a grounding pad. This allows for deep penetration and was initially utilized in electrosurgery. Safety concerns and high pain levels may be associated with this type of device.[3] Bipolar describes a system in which electric current moves between two electrodes at the surface of an intended treatment site. Compared with monopolar systems, they are more limited in the depth they can achieve, which is approximately half the distance between two electrodes (Fig. 7.2).[1,3]

Groups that have marketed RF devices for fat reduction have taken technology several steps further. Pollogen® Ltd (Tel Aviv, Israel) has developed a line of RF devices with three electrodes, referred to as TriPollar® technology. In this design, current flows from one positive to two independent negative electrodes (Fig. 7.3) to produce uniform but relatively deep heating.[7] Both the Regen XL™ and Apollo™ devices emit a frequency of 1 MHz at 30 to 50 W and have been shown to have destructive effects on adipocytes. Boisnic and Branchet performed an ex vivo study on 12 skin samples from eight abdominoplasty patients treated locally with the Apollo™ device (50 W). They reported an increased glycerol level from the hypodermis of treated skin (5610.2 nm/g) compared to untreated skin (2549.4 nm/g) suggesting increased lipolysis in treated skin. Of the skin samples they evaluated histologically, two of four showed inhomogeneity of adipocyte membranes, which were elongated and irregular at some sectors with partial rupture of cell walls. One sample showed a necrotic area of adipocytes. These results suggest direct effects of RF on adipocyte membrane integrity (Fig. 7.4).[8] In a second trial, an at-home tripolar device showed similar increased glycerol release in eight skin samples compared with controls: 4180.8 nM/g vs 2301.8 nM/g. In the same study, 34% of adipocytes were modified in shape with inhomogeneity, elongation, irregularity and membrane changes including partial rupture. Unfortunately, the study was limited in that it did not report the percentage of change in untreated tissue.[9] Finally, Kaplan and Gat demonstrated similar changes to adipocytes in a patient treated with the Regen™ device (30 W). This patient consented to histologic analysis following seven weekly treatments. Dermal thickness increased by 49% compared with untreated skin, though thickness of the subcutaneous

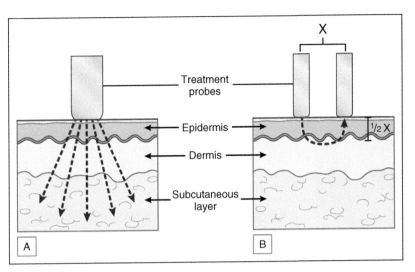

Figure 7.2 (A) Monopolar radiofrequency device. **(B)** Bipolar radiofrequency device

layer appeared unchanged between treated and untreated skin.[10]

Histologic changes in adipocytes have been reported with additional RF technologies. Trelles et al. employed an automatic multi-frequency and low impedance RF device (ThermaLipo™, Thermamedic Ltd, Alicante, Spain), which emits at a lower frequency (0.6 MHz) to target deeper tissues and at higher frequency (2.4 MHz) for more superficial tissue. Thirty women were treated with this device at the buttocks for at least four passes in order to reach a skin temperature of 42 °C maintained for a minimum of 12 minutes. Skin biopsies were taken prior to and 2 hours after RF treatment and stained with H&E and Oil red O separately. In all samples, adipocytes lost their typically round shape and became more polyhedric and rectangular. Degeneration of the cellular membrane was observed as well as vacuolization of fat and decreased fat. Some cells appeared necrotic.[11]

Pearl 2

Effective radiofrequency fat reduction requires that the skin is maintained at ≈40–42 °C for several minutes and multiple passes. Since fat is a good insulator, the temperature of the skin may not always be an indicator of fat temperature. A series of treatments may provide improved results.

Another recent and unique RF design includes an applicator consisting of a series of tightly spaced concentric rings that are designed to couple energy into tissue across the entire surface of the applicator (truSculpt™, Cutera®, Brisbane, CA) (Fig. 7.5). The distribution of surface electric potential is controlled by adjusting frequency to create uniform heating at specified volumes. Electric fields are created in a perpendicular manner to the dermal–subcutaneous junction resulting in significant, targeted heating of the fat. This was demonstrated in two subjects in whom temperature probes were inserted at the cutaneous–subcutaneous junction, 7 mm into the subcutaneous tissue, and 12 mm into the subcutaneous tissue during general anesthesia induced for planned abdominoplasty. The truSculpt device was applied for 3 minutes and probes reported that the temperature of the cutaneous–subcutaneous junction remained <30 °C while the temperatures at 7 mm and 12 mm reached 45 °C and 50 °C, respectively.[5] Resulting subcutaneous changes are shown by another phase of the same study in which three patients were treated for 22 minutes prior to abdominoplasty and then underwent biopsies of the treated sites. Epidermal and dermal structures were normal in all biopsies and the subcutaneous tissue appeared normal immediately after the procedure. Yet, beginning at day 4, adipose tissue showed vascular alterations including purpura, congested vessels and increased vascularity. Adipocyte necrosis was noted at day 9 in one patient and at days 17 and 24 in a second patient while increased macrophages and foamy histiocytes were noted on day 10 in a third patient. The authors suggest that fat is disposed of and therefore volumetrically decreased by phagocytosis in a gradual manner that does not lead to hyperlipidemia.[5]

Several body contouring devices that emit RF actually induce a field of low level, nonionizing radiation. The Accent® family of devices produced by Alma Lasers™ (Buffalo Grove, IL) includes a unipolar device, which Emilia del Pino et al. and Goldberg et al. have described.[12,13] It is marketed as a device to improve the appearance of cellulite, as are many body contouring RF devices, but has demonstrated measurable dimensional change to subcutaneous tissue and decreased thigh circumference.[12,13]

The Vanquish™ (BTL Aesthetics, Prague, CR) system emits RF over a large field and is being called focused field RF. This novel device has its origins in diathermy treatment, which is a deep heating form of treatment for muscle soreness. While relatively independent of an operator, it requires movement of the large RF field delivery

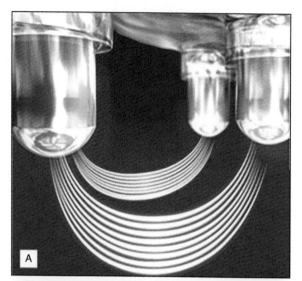

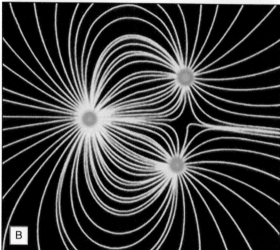

Figure 7.3 TriPollar® technology *(from Manuskiatti W, et al. Circumference reduction and cellulite treatment with a TriPollar radiofrequency device: a pilot study. J Eur Acad Dermatol Venereol 2009; 23(7):820–7, with permission from Pollogen)*

nuclei and demonstrated an apoptotic index of 52/100, increased from 13/100 prior to treatment. Histologic evaluation of treated areas showed disrupted adipocytes and gross pathology demonstrated a clear decrease in subcutaneous tissue (Fig. 7.7).[6] A recent study by Fajkosova et al.[14] supports the idea that this technology is effective in humans as well. In a study of 40 people, 35 of whom completed the study, there was a mean decrease in abdominal circumference of 4.93 cm after four weekly treatments of 30 minutes. There were only three nonresponders and it was postulated that the technology was not successful in these patients because they represented the slimmest subjects with the least subcutaneous tissue.[14]

Patient selection

Careful patient selection is important for successful fat reduction with RF devices. Overall body habitus is an important consideration as most of these devices are unlikely to be effective in patients who are grossly overweight or obese. For instance, the truSculpt is recommended for individuals with a BMI between 22 and 28.[15] RF body contouring devices are not designed as weight reduction tools or as substitutes for liposuction or gastric bypass/bandage.[16] In overweight individuals, the resulting reduction in adiposity will not be appreciable and, since these devices are currently designed to target subcutaneous fat, they are unlikely to have an effect on deeper abdominal fat. An exception to this rule is the Vanquish device, which is more useful in overweight individuals due to its large treatment head. Patients with close-to-desired body weight and discrete areas of undesired fatty tissue, such as those located at love handles, buttocks, and thighs, are generally good candidates. A simple bedside test is to determine if a patient's undesired fat may be grasped or pinched. If so, it is more likely cutaneous and amenable to RF treatment. The caveat being that pinched tissue should be greater than 1–2 cm in width to ensure that undesired areas do in fact contain excess adiposity rather than just epidermal and dermal tissue.

head and is contactless (Fig. 7.6). The large delivery head allows treatment of relatively obese patients, even those with BMIs between 30 and 35. It is designed to deliver energy to tissue with a specific impedance, taking advantage of the water content of tissue with more resistance and heat created in tissue with less water content. Fat has less water content and therefore heats up relative to surrounding skin and muscle. In the US, it is currently FDA-approved for deep tissue heating but also seems to reduce fat due to adipocyte damage. In an animal study using four Vietnamese pigs, the Vanquish RF applicator was placed 1 cm above the skin for a total of 30 minutes during which the skin temperature was maintained between 39 °C and 42 °C. This was done four times. At the end of treatment, the TUNEL method was employed to detect apoptotic

Pearl 3

One bedside test to determine whether a patient is a candidate for radiofrequency fat reduction technology is to attempt to grasp or pinch their unwanted fat. Deeper abdominal fat that is not graspable is unlikely to improve with these subcutaneous-directed modalities. The Vanquish device is an exception and may be useful in overweight individuals.

In general, appropriate candidates are in good overall health.[15,16] Any skin type may be treated with RF making it more widely applicable than some laser systems which cannot safely be used on darker skin types. These devices have not been studied in children and may not be appropriate for those under the age of 18. Fortunately, side effects are limited and downtime is minimal, making RF

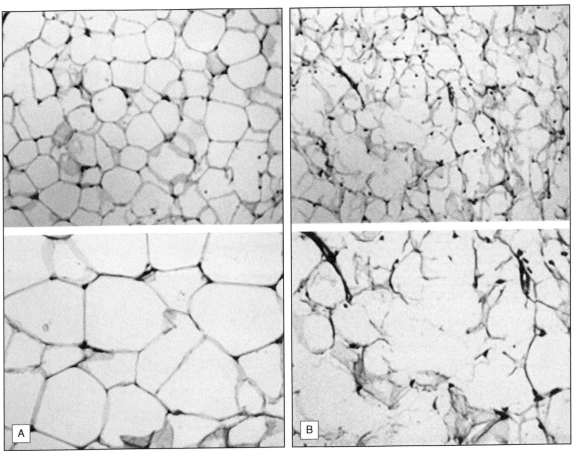

Figure 7.4 (A) Subcutaneous tissue prior to treatment. **(B)** Subcutaneous tissue following radiofrequency treatment showing polyhedric cells and membrane degeneration *(with permission from Pollogen)*

Box 7.1
Characteristics of preferred radiofrequency fat reduction candidates

- Good overall health
- Adults greater than 18 years of age
- Patients of all skin types
- BMI between 22 and 28 (includes patients already at preferred body weight; exception is patients undergoing the Vanquish™ procedure)
- Discrete areas of graspable cutaneous fat at least 1–2 cm in thickness
- Problem areas that include the abdomen, love handles, and thighs
- Problem areas **do not** include deeper visceral fat

Typical treatment course

The expected treatment course and recommended protocol varies between devices. However, all treatment strategies involve heating the adipose tissue to a goal temperature range ($\approx$40–45 °C) for a specific length of time and generally a series of treatments is recommended (Table 7.1). The most likely side effect following these procedures is erythema lasting up to 2–3 hours at the site of treatment. In general, the procedures should not be particularly painful. Rather, the sensation of a warm massage is often experienced with the more common direct-contact devices. In a small study of four subjects, patients reported that the contactless Vanquish procedure was either comfortable or very comfortable.[17]

interventions feasible for those with busy schedules. Another group that may be particularly well suited for these procedures are those patients who wish to avoid more invasive surgical procedures that present a less favorable side effect profile and result in increased downtime (Box 7.1).

Pearl 4

When using radiofrequency handpieces, slow rotating movements with slight pressure will make the heating of skin more tolerable to patients.

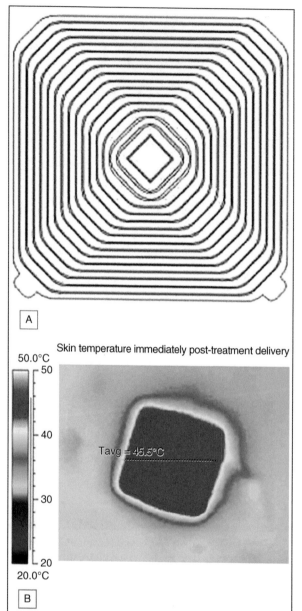

Figure 7.5 (A) Ventral surface of the truSculpt applicator, showing a series of tightly spaced concentric rings. **(B)** Skin temperature immediately post-treatment. The device is designed to deliver uniform heating at the skin's surface *(with permission from truSculpt)*

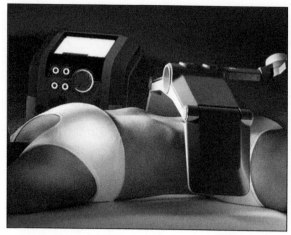

Figure 7.6 Vanquish device

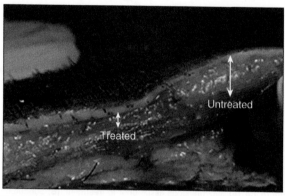

Figure 7.7 Gross pathology of the skin of Vietnamese pig treated with the Vanquish device. Note the decreased height of subcutaneous tissue in treated skin (left side) compared to untreated skin (right side)

Pollogen recommends that TriPollar devices (1 MHz) be utilized for courses of 4–8 treatments that are no less than 1 week apart. Each treatment lasts 20–40 minutes and is essentially pain free. During the treatment, glycerin is applied to the skin to prevent overheating of the epidermis. The clinician rotates a handpiece on the skin using slight pressure with a goal skin temperature of 40–42 °C for several minutes. Handpieces come in small, medium and large sizes with the latter being best suited for the abdomen, flanks, thighs, and buttocks. Patients may return to their daily routines immediately following the procedure.[18]

The unipolar Accent device (40 MHz) treatments, which are marketed as improving the appearance of cellulite, last for up to 45 minutes and are repeated at 2-week intervals for 3–5 treatments. Again, a handpiece is rubbed with slight pressure against the target treatment sites. During the study by Goldberg et al., this was done using an applicator with a cooling tip for 30 seconds for three passes with skin reaching 40–42 °C.[13] Patients may describe the sensation of the treatment as a warm massage and erythema should persist no more than 24 hours.[19]

Pearl 5

Pain is minimal with radiofrequency fat-reducing procedures and patients may return to their normal routines immediately. They should be counseled to expect treatment-related erythema for no more than 24 hours.

Table 7.1 Recommended treatment guidelines for selected RF fat reduction technologies

Device	Individual treatment length	Recommended number of treatments	Frequency of treatments
TriPollar® Pollogen®, Tel Aviv, Israel	20–40 minutes	4–8	≥1 week
truSculpt™ Cutera®, Brisbane, CA	< 60 minutes	2–4	4–8 weeks
Accent® family Alma Lasers, Buffalo Grove, IL	≤ 45 minutes	3–5	2 weeks
Vanquish™ BTL Aesthetics, Prague, CR	30 minutes	4	weekly

In the truSculpt protocol, 2–4 treatments are recommended at 4–8-week intervals. Each treatment takes less than an hour with individual pulse durations lasting 4 minutes. Pain should be rated at no more than approximately 4 out of 10 and may improve as patients become used to the sensation as a treatment progresses. With this device, patients may tolerate a skin temperature of up to 45 °C. Erythema is expected for several hours following the procedure.[20]

Patients utilizing the Vanquish device undergo a series of four treatments lasting 30 minutes each. This procedure is unique in that the device does not come into contact with the patient. Rather, a curved arm extends from the machine and hovers over the patient during the treatment protocol. The procedure is painless and patients experience a mild to moderate heat sensation.[21]

Expected results

Results may be difficult to predict as RF devices are dependent on tissue impedance, which varies from person to person based on individual composition of adipose tissue. Furthermore, the data demonstrating the clinical efficacy of these devices remains in its infancy and, in some instances, is conflicting between studies. A common measurement used to demonstrate efficacy is circumference. Unfortunately, this efficacy measurement mechanism is only a substitute for fat reduction and does not necessarily reflect a decreased subcutaneous layer. For instance, decreased circumference may also result from overall tissue tightening or even decreased edema following some interventions that include massage. Other modalities that may provide more insight include ultrasound measurements of the distance from dermis to muscle and, in some cases, tissue evaluation by biopsy.

Levenberg reported 37 patients undergoing between 2 and 15 weekly treatments with the TriPollar Apollo™ device emitting at 1 MHz for a maximum of 50 W. There were statistically significant changes in abdomen, buttocks and thigh circumference with decreases of 4.5 cm, 3.1 cm, and 2.4 cm, respectively.[22] Though measurements were taken in a uniform fashion prior to and after treatment,

no other measurements of the subcutaneous layer that utilized imaging (i.e. ultrasound) or histopathologic evaluation were utilized. Manuskiatti and colleagues reported on the similar TriPollar Regen® device, which was used at 1 MHz for 20–28.5 W and a skin temperature of 40–42 °C. The statistically significant average decreases of 3.5 cm and 1.7 cm in abdominal and thigh circumference, respectively, were reported in 21 patients (per treatment site). There was no change in buttocks or arm circumference.[7] Using ultrasound measurements, they also reported a statistically significant decrease in distance from epidermis to superficial fascia at the thighs, averaging 0.61 mm.[7] Unfortunately, this is an extremely small value and does not rule out a change in dermal dimensions rather than subcutaneous dimensions. Interestingly, patients' weights also decreased by an average of 0.69 kg, which slightly confounds the results, making it possible that circumference changes were secondary to weight loss rather than the treatment. This does not exclude the possibility that the weight loss could have been secondary to the treatment.

Mlosek et al. described 45 women undergoing a controlled study with a tripolar device by Beauty Light Science and Technology Co., Ltd (Beijing, China). This device was designed to improve the appearance of cellulite. Yet, using ultrasound, it was also shown that subcutaneous tissue at the thigh decreased a statistically significant amount from 17.152 cm to 14.924 cm after eight weekly procedures. Thigh circumference also decreased from 56.375 cm to 54.286 cm. Placebo groups showed no statistical change in either category. This study is limited in part by its method of measurement as ultrasound can provide dimensional information regarding subcutaneous tissue but it cannot describe whether the quality and/or quantity of adipocytes was actually affected.[23]

In del Pino's study, the thighs and buttocks of 26 women were treated with a unipolar high-energy device designed to reach depths of 2 cm at 150 W (40.68 MHz) for three passes of 30 seconds and skin temperatures of 39–41 °C. There were two sessions, 15 days apart. Using ultrasound to measure the distance from the dermal–epidermal junction to Camper's fascia, 72% of patients

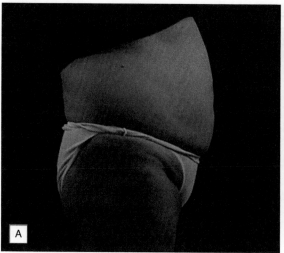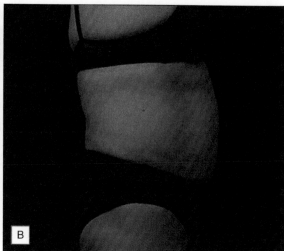

Figure 7.8 (A) Before and **(B)** after treatment with the Vanquish™ device

showed an average reduction of 2.64 mm (27%) at the thighs and 64% of patients showed an average reduction of 1.8 mm at the buttocks.[12] These results are not marked and p-values were not reported.[12] It should also be noted that Goldberg et al., who studied a similar unipolar device at the thighs in 30 women, did not show a lasting decreased distance from dermis to Camper's fascia 6 months after treatment.[13] In this study, there were a total of six sessions performed every other week with an Accent device at 150–170 W for three passes of 30 seconds, reaching a skin temperature of 40–42 °C. Thigh circumference was measured prior to treatment and 6 months post-treatment. The mean decrease was 2.45 cm in 27 of 30 patients and leg smoothness improvement on a 1 to 4 scale was noted as 2.9.[13]

In an early report regarding the Vanquish device, five patients were treated with the noncontact technology for four treatments reaching a maximum of 170 W. Three of four patients showed circumferential reduction at the abdomen/love handle area of 5 cm on average (Fig. 7.8)[17] A more recent study by Fajkosova et al. supports that this technology is effective. In a report of 40 people, 35 of whom completed the study, there was a mean decrease in abdominal circumference of 4.93 cm after four weekly treatments of 30 minutes. There were only three nonresponders and it was postulated that the technology was not successful in these patients because they represented the slimmest subjects with the least amount of subcutaneous tissue.[14]

The efficacy of RF for fat reduction may be modest. Further investigation with larger trials and long-term follow-up greater than 6 months would be beneficial to provide more accurate and useful data.

Safety

Safety profiles should certainly be considered for individual technologies; but overall, RF devices rarely cause short- or long-term adverse events. Post-procedure erythema lasting several hours is to be expected.[7] Erythematous papules, papular urticaria, first degree burns, blisters and bruising have been reported with the Regen Tripollar device. This was likely secondary to excessively slow movement of the handpiece and an inadequate amount of glycerin oil and these side effects were generally mild, asymptomatic and self-limited.[7] Goldberg and colleagues found no blistering, scarring or pigment changes when using the Accent unipolar system and no changes in blood lipids were noted.[13] Similarly, Levenberg reported no significant changes in liver function tests or lipid analysis performed in five patients following two treatments with the Apollo TriPollar device.[22] No adverse events have been reported secondary to Vanquish.

Multimodality procedures

Recently, RF has been employed as a single modality treatment for fat reduction. However, a combined bipolar RF, infrared (IR), and suction massage device (VelaShape™, Syneron® Medical Ltd) should be mentioned as it is the only FDA-approved device for circumferential reduction of the thigh. In 2005, Alster and Tanzi reported that in 20 women treated with this device, the average reduction in thigh circumference was 0.8 cm. This was noted after eight biweekly treatments during which the device was set to emit 20 W of RF, 20 W of IR (700–1500 nm) light, and 750 mmHg negative pressure. It is likely that this multi-modality intervention is similarly effective as other RF fat reduction devices.

Conclusion

Noninvasive body contouring techniques have become a staple cosmetic procedure. They represent low risk interventions with little downtime that many patients with discrete areas of unwanted fat may safely utilize. RF devices have long been a mainstay for contouring procedures, particularly skin tightening, and may now be employed for fat reduction. Technology in this area is rapidly progressing from classic monopolar and bipolar machines to those which utilize tripolar technology, contactless nonionizing radiation, and handpieces that induce uniform electric fields with tight concentric ring-shaped electrodes. While the mechanism(s) of action may be somewhat unclear, it is evident by histologic examination that adipocytes are susceptible to RF-induced bulk heating. Data is somewhat sparse regarding the efficacy of these devices, but this lack of literature represents an avenue that remains open for further research and innovation.

CASE STUDY 1

A 40-year-old male presents to clinic with the complaint of bilateral love handles. Despite regular exercise and a healthy diet, he cannot eliminate these specific areas of fatty deposition.

On clinical examination, he demonstrates classic fat hypertrophy at the bilateral lateral and posterior waistline, which may be grasped for approximately 3 cm of width.

Lipodystrophy located at the love handles is an excellent condition to be treated for fat reduction by radiofrequency technology. This patient, who has very localized and resistant depositions of fat, should respond beautifully to any of the radiofrequency devices, including the TriPollar, truSculpt, Accent and Vanquish devices. Between two and eight treatments will be necessary depending on the chosen device (see Table 7.1).

CASE STUDY 2

A 50-year-old female with a body mass index of 33 presents with the complaint of excess fatty tissue at the abdomen and flanks. She admits that she is somewhat overweight but has difficulty maintaining a regular exercise schedule and has not been able to change her shape.

On physical examination she exhibits increased fat deposition at the upper and lower abdomen and the flanks bilaterally. The width of the fatty layer upon grasping is >5 cm.

This obese woman may not be an excellent candidate for very localized forms of radiofrequency treatment but should respond well to the Vanquish technology. At least four visits, each lasting 30 minutes, should be planned.

References

1. Lolis MS, Goldberg DJ. Radiofrequency in cosmetic dermatology: a review. Dermatol Surg 2012;38(11):1765–76.
2. Atiyeh BS, Dibo SA. Nonsurgical nonablative treatment of aging skin: radiofrequency technologies between aggressive marketing and evidence-based efficacy. Aesthetic Plast Surg 2009;33(3):283–94.
3. Bogle MA. Radiofrequency energy and hybrid devices. In: Alam M, Jeffrey S, editors. Non-surgical skin tightening and lifting. Elsevier; 2009. p. 21–32.
4. Franco W, Kothare A, Goldberg DJ. Controlled volumetric heating of subcutaneous adipose tissue using a novel radiofrequency technology. Lasers Surg Med 2009; 41(10):745–50.
5. Franco W, Kothare A, Ronan SJ, et al. Hyperthermic injury to adipocyte cells by selective heating of subcutaneous fat with a novel radiofrequency device: feasibility studies. Lasers Surg Med 2010;42(5):361–70.
6. Weiss R, Weiss M, Beasley K, et al. Operator independent focused high frequency ISM band for fat reduction: porcine model. Lasers Surg Med 2013;45(4):235–9.
7. Manuskiatti W, Wachirakaphan C, Lektrakul N, Varothai S. Circumference reduction and cellulite treatment with a TriPollar radiofrequency device: a pilot study. J Eur Acad Dermatol Venereol 2009;23(7):820–7.
8. Boisnic S, Branchet MC. Ex vivo human skin evaluation of localized fat reduction and anti-aging effect by TriPollar radio frequency treatments. J Cosmet Laser Ther 2010;12(1): 25–31.
9. Boisnic S, Branchet MC, Birnstiel O, Beilin G. Clinical and histopathological study of the TriPollar home-use device for body treatments. Eur J Dermatol 2010;20(3):367–72.
10. Kaplan H, Gat A. Clinical and histopathological results following TriPollar radiofrequency skin treatments. J Cosmet Laser Ther 2009;11(2):78–84.
11. Trelles MA, van der Lugt C, Mordon S, et al. Histological findings in adipocytes when cellulite is treated with a variable-emission radiofrequency system. Lasers Med Sci 2010;25(2):191–5.
12. Emilia del Pino M, Rosado RH, Azuela A, et al. Effect of controlled volumetric tissue heating with radiofrequency on cellulite and the subcutaneous tissue of the buttocks and thighs. J Drugs Dermatol 2006 5(8):714–22.
13. Goldberg DJ, Fazeli A, Berlin AL. Clinical, laboratory, and MRI analysis of cellulite treatment with a unipolar radiofrequency device. Dermatol Surg 2008;34(2):204–9, discussion 209.
14. Fajkosova K, Machovcova A, Onder M, Fritz K. Selective radiofrequency therapy as a non-invasive approach for contactless body contouring and circumferential reduction. J Drugs Dermatol 2014;13(3):291–6.
15. Cutera. Introducing the truSculpt System. 2012.
16. BTL Aesthetics. Online (cited January 11 2014). Available: <http://www.btlvanquish.com/en/for-physicians.html>.
17. Fajkosova K, Machovcova A, Fritz K. Selective RF therapy as a non-invasive approach for contactless body contouring and circumferential reduction. Preliminary case report. Cosmet Med 2013;34.
18. Pollogen. Customer FAQs. Online (cited 19 January 2014). Available: <http://www.pollogen.com/patients/patient-faqs.html>.
19. Alma Lasers. The accent experience. Online (cited 19 January 2014). Available: <http://www.accentyourbody.com/pages/accent_experience.html>.
20. Cutera. Patient FAQs. Online (cited 19 January 2014). Available: <trusculpt.com/faq.php>.
21. BTL Aesthetics. Reveal the Vanquish World. Online (11 January 2014). Available: <http://www.btlvanquish.com/en/faqs.html>.
22. Levenberg A. Clinical experience with a TriPollar radiofrequency system for facial and body aesthetic treatments. Eur J Dermatol 2010;20(5):615–19.
23. Mlosek RK, Wozniak W, Malinowska S, et al. The effectiveness of anticellulite treatment using tripolar radiofrequency monitored by classic and high-frequency ultrasound. J Eur Acad Dermatol Venereol 2012;26(6):696–703.

Ultrasound Treatment: Fat Reduction

8

Mark L. Jewell, Deanne M. Robinson,
James L. Jewell

Key Messages

- The demand for noninvasive body sculpting procedures is on the rise
- High intensity focused ultrasound (HIFU) offers a noninvasive alternative for body contouring
- HIFU is FDA cleared for the reduction of waist circumference
- HIFU treatment is indicated for treatment of localized collections of subcutaneous adipose tissue resistant to diet and exercise
- A single HIFU treatment of the abdomen and flanks generally produces a >2 cm reduction in waist circumference

Introduction/proposed mechanism of action

Ultrasonic energy is used in medicine for a variety of applications, imaging, physical therapy, and tissue ablation. The focus of this chapter is to explore the use of high intensity focused ultrasound (HIFU) in noninvasive body contouring. HIFU is an ablative therapy, producing thermal damage to targeted tissue. Tissue thermodynamics, dosimetry, and mode of HIFU application are relevant for the successful use of HIFU to achieve tissue ablation for therapeutic or cosmetic outcomes.

Simply, sonic energy can be focused like light, according to the design of the transducer. Unfocused sonic energy can pass through skin and structures above and below the focal zone in fluence levels low enough to not produce substantive tissue heating. Yet within the focus zone, tissue can be rapidly heated to 55–65 °C, which will produce thermal necrosis. This rapid temperature rise affects all structures within the target zone, including tissue layers that involve subcutaneous adipose tissue (SAT) that is rich in collagen. Type I collagen will undergo denaturation and shrinkage at approximately 65 °C to 70 °C, a temperature far too high for tissue survival.[1-5] Once denaturation occurs, a biologic response to wounding proceeds.[6]

Biologic response to heating has been studied either by prolonged static exposure to heat or in terms of a temperature jump where tissue reaction (damage) rates relate to an Arrhenius equation.[7-9] The transfer of heat into tissues has been quantified by the Pennes bioheat equation and finite element modeling.[9,10] There has been meaningful experimental work done to understand the nature of thermal burns and the response of tissue to heating.[11-15] Full thickness skin burns have been produced with skin temperatures in the 47 °C range in animals.[11] Thermal damage to skin is thought to occur as low as 44 °C.[16] Skin blood flow ceases at approximately 45 °C.[10] If the thermal response of tissue necrosis is plotted, there is a break in the slope of the curve at 43 °C in terms of a dramatic decrease in exposure time required to produce skin necrosis.[9] There is little margin for error in heating tissue at near-burn levels, when it is possible to transition to irreversible thermal damage very rapidly.

The lesions produced with HIFU in deeper layers are referred to as 'trackless lesions' because tissue ablation only occurs within the focal zone.[17] High-amplitude millimeter wavelength ultrasound is focused within clinically relevant tissue volumes. Ultrasound propagates through the aqueous medium that comprises most of the human body. Depending on the tissue type, there can be attenuation of the energy. Within the focal zone, part of the mechanical energy carried by the incident wave is converted into heat by viscous absorption. This constitutes the primary mechanism for ultrasound-induced hyperthermia (thermal ultrasound). Frequencies near 1 MHz appear most effective for tissue heating. Lower frequencies of 500 kHz work best for deeper heating and higher frequencies in the 8 MHz range work optimally for more superficial heating.[17] Another consideration is the need for deliberate avoidance of cavitation within the target zone, as the presence of microbubbles dramatically changes tissue impedance and causes energy reflection and dissipation.

Besides energy production and focusing, dosimetry and patterns of energy delivery are relevant to producing the uniform tissue heating required for a cosmetic or therapeutic effect. When using HIFU to ablate SAT, the improvement in body contour occurs due to volume loss of ablated fat, thermal modulation and remodeling of collagen, and passive skin tightening due to undersurface volume reduction over time.

In the case of the Liposonix® device (Solta Medical Inc., Hayward, CA), when focused into tissues, HIFU produces a lesion about the size of a grain of rice. The microprocessor-controlled transducer is moved through a grid pattern to produce an 'X by Y' zone of lesions. There are parallels between what is occurring with this device and fractional lasers, where a small proportion of the tissue within the treatment zone receives energy. This approach avoids excess bulk heating and ensuing thermal damage (e.g. skin burns, damage to collateral structures, or fat necrosis). By leaving intact tissue around lesions, blood supply is not compromised and macrophages can start removal of tissue debris and extracellular lipid within the treated SAT. Other forms of unfocused ultrasound produce a tissue effect in deeper layers by bulk heating. Adipocytes respond by releasing lipid, but are not destroyed.

Thus, the HIFU device provides a means to produce fractional ablation of SAT and thermally modulate collagen at a focal zone 13–26 mm below the epidermis. Following a HIFU treatment, a mild inflammatory response occurs, with macrophage infiltration.[18] Cellular debris and extracellular lipid are removed and metabolized in the liver; collagen within the mid-lamellar matrix (MLM) that has been subjected to thermal heating remodels and tightens. Very soon after treatment, tissue haziness associated with extracellular lipid is noted on diagnostic ultrasound (DUS). The net clinical effect following the wound healing cascade is an internal 'shrink wrap' effect within the treatment zone. A 12–16-week period is required to achieve this final outcome.[19,20]

The initial pre-clinical research performed with the Liposonix device determined that optimal tissue response required between 140 and 180 J/cm^2. Higher energy dosing did not produce a superior clinical outcome.[18] During treatment, a 5×5 cm grid that approximates the size of the transducer is drawn around each treatment zone. Water is used as the coupling agent between the plastic window of the transducer assembly called the replaceable treatment cartridge (RTC). Transducer assemblies have finite lifespans and are replaced after approximately 6000 firings.

The approach for energy delivery consists of treating a zone and then moving on to the next treatment zone ('grid repeat'). The process is repeated as often as appropriate, according to the fluence setting of the HIFU device. Alternatively, a second approach involves the repeated firing of the RTC within the same zone, as tolerated by the patient ('site stacking'). This approach, while more time-efficient, may produce discomfort and a feeling of excess warmth within the deeper tissues, depending on fluence level. An advantage of site stacking is that treatment can be modified with lower fluences that maximize patient comfort.

Pre-clinical research with HIFU in pigs did not show collateral damage to blood vessels that were in the region of the treatment zone. That being said, cutaneous nerves within the treatment area may be irritated and inflamed with HIFU, given the large amount of lipid found within the myelin sheath. This phenomenon has been noted with ultrasonic-assisted lipoplasty devices. Dysesthesias can

occur and are self-limiting. It would be theoretically possible to damage major nerve trunks if HIFU was applied to anatomic areas where these structures are located (inner arm, sub-gluteal banana roll, and posterior thigh).

Inflammatory fat necrosis from bulk tissue heating may occur with laser-assisted liposuction. Photomicrographs of laser-treated SAT show inflammatory fat necrosis and vascular occlusion[21] but such necrosis has not been encountered in the Liposonix pre-clinical and pivotal studies. There is the possibility that inflammatory fat necrosis could develop if sufficient tissue heating were to occur, but this potential risk is minimized when HIFU is administered in a fractional approach.

HIFU for fat reduction is a novel therapy that will be further refined in the future. Future HIFU devices may combine both real-time imaging and shear wave elastography imaging to track and optimize treatment effectiveness. Additionally, a variable focus HIFU/RTC apparatus may permit more shallow treatment zones, including treatment of the dermis alone. HIFU may also be combined with other energy-emitting devices such as radiofrequency. Indeed, far downstream there is the possibility that HIFU may supplant ionizing radiation for the treatment of malignancies.

Patient selection

HIFU for fat reduction is a noninvasive body sculpting modality cleared by the FDA for circumferential waist reduction. This method is an alternative for selected patients who are unable to undergo, or would like to avoid, more invasive procedures, such as traditional liposuction. Pilot and confirmatory studies reveal that HIFU treatment of the flanks and abdomen consistently produces a greater than 2 cm reduction in abdominal circumference after a single treatment. In consultation with potential patients, clear expectations of post-treatment results should be extensively discussed and reviewed. It should also be made clear that HIFU is a body contouring procedure and is not indicated for weight reduction or treatment of obesity.

Pearl 1

Appropriate patient selection and thorough discussion of expected outcomes are imperative for patient satisfaction.

Ideal candidates for HIFU treatment are individuals with a localized collection of SAT of the abdomen or flanks that has proven resistant to conventional diet and exercise. Ideal patient characteristics include BMI<30, good skin tone and elasticity, at least 2.5 cm of SAT in the desired treatment area, a treatment zone free of scars, and realistic outcome expectations (Box 8.1). In evaluation of potential patients, the pinch test or calipers can be used to evaluate SAT volume. To additionally verify and quantify the thickness of SAT, a DUS may be utilized.

Box 8.1
Ideal patient characteristics

- BMI < 30
- Good skin tone and elasticity
- >2.5 cm of SAT in the desired treatment area
- Free of scars within the treatment zone
- Realistic outcome expectations

Box 8.2
Contraindications to HIFU treatment

- Hernia in the treatment area
- Pregnant females or females suspected to be pregnant
- <1 cm of SAT in the treatment zone

Pearl 2

Ideal HIFU candidates have: BMI<30, good skin tone, and >2.5 cm of SAT in the desired treatment areas.

Contraindications to HIFU treatment include hernia in the treatment area, pregnancy or possible pregnancy, and less than 1 cm of SAT in the treatment zone (Box 8.2). Other relative contraindications for HIFU treatment include active systemic illnesses, therapeutic anticoagulation, history of thromboembolic disease, implanted metal or electronic devices, or severe hepatic disease. As such, a thorough medical history and physical examination should be performed prior to treatment.

Pearl 3

Contraindications to HIFU treatment are pregnancy, or hernia within the treatment area.

Pain tolerance is another important patient factor to be considered before treatment initiation. Solish et al.[24] report that the vast majority (90%) of patients undergoing HIFU treatment received pre-treatment analgesia with oral opiates. Procedure-associated pain was rated as minimal to mild for the majority of subjects receiving treatment with 47 J/cm^2, 52 J/cm^2, and 59 J/cm^2, and only two patients required additional intraoperative analgesia. There was a trend towards increased procedure associated discomfort in the higher fluence group, with patients in the 59 J/cm^2 group experiencing the greatest discomfort. However, this difference did not reach statistical significance. Similar procedure-associated pain was reported by Jewell et al.[20] Of the treated patients, 22% of patients received pre-, intra-, or post-procedure analgesic (acetaminophen, ibuprofen, or naproxen), and most patients reported mild to moderate procedural discomfort. In the 47 and 59 J/cm^2 groups, 5.1% and 9.5% of subjects, respectively, reported severe procedural pain,

thus echoing the observation made by Solish of increased pain with higher fluence treatments. There were no reports of severe post-procedural pain and all mild to moderate pain resolved within 7–10 days. Thus, providers may choose to have a candid conversation with prospective patients regarding their pain tolerance in order to ensure appropriate analgesia.

Pearl 4

Individualized attention to pre-, intra-, and post-treatment pain management will optimize procedure outcomes.

Typical treatment course

The concept of noninvasive body contouring procedures is particularly attractive to patients who seek to achieve a modest improvement in body contour without an invasive surgical procedure and the associated downtime. In order to evaluate patients for HIFU treatment, an understanding of body morphology and laminar anatomy is needed.

The human body has a variety of superficial tissue layers: skin; superficial fat; collagen-rich MLM; deep fat; and deep fascia (overlying muscles such as the rectus abdominis). Factors which influence the degree of fat deposition in each of the layers include genetics, gender, and BMI, as well as recent weight gain or loss. Various technologies target fat in specific layers. Cryolipolysis appears to work best on fat in the superficial to MLM compartments, provided that such regions can be sandwiched into the device handpiece. Because it is a cold-subtraction technology, cryolipolysis may be less likely to tighten collagen like the thermal HIFU technologies.

HIFU body contouring technologies work best with a relatively thicker layer of SAT because of their ability to focus energy into the MLM. Individuals with skin to deep fascia of ≈2.3 cm appear to achieve good results. Individuals with thinner SAT find HIFU treatments to be uncomfortable because the HIFU energy hits the deep fascia. Those with thicker layers and elevated BMI have too much superficial fat thickness, which prevents the HIFU from reaching the collagen-rich MLM where fat reduction and thermal modulation of collagen can occur. Other very thin individuals have tissue thickness primarily in the MLM, with inadequate overall tissue layer thickness for HIFU as it exists currently. These individuals are also poor candidates for liposuction due to the very fibrous nature of the MLM. In summary, two requisite conditions must exist for an optimal HIFU treatment candidate: BMI < 30 and skin to deep fascia measurements of approximately 2.3 cm. Most patients in this realm have a clearly demarcated start of the MLM at about 11 mm beneath the skin on DUS imaging.[22]

Having a DUS machine available for the screening of patients seeking noninvasive body contouring can be helpful. DUS can accurately measure tissue to deep fascia depth. This determines suitability for HIFU treatment, conventional liposuction, or polite counseling regarding a weight loss program of diet, exercise, and lifestyle modification. Liposonix and other forms of noninvasive body contouring should not be viewed as an 'all-comers' type of body contouring.

Other important considerations for patient selection are adequate skin tone, absence of loose or hanging skin, and an adequate patient focus on fitness, weight, and lifestyle. Those who do not monitor their personal weight tend to have weight fluctuations that interfere with obtaining the best result with noninvasive body contouring procedures. Careful documentation of waist circumferences (e.g. precision measurement with a laser level device and spring-loaded measuring tape) may thus be an integral part of patient evaluation. Even in situations of diminished skin tone and elasticity in the post-menopausal female, change in waistline circumference can be produced with HIFU in patients who otherwise would not be considered for liposuction. Alternatively, excisional body contouring procedures, such as lipoabdominoplasty, remain the best option when there are loose tissues, diminished skin tone, and deep layer laxity.

The use of simple data templates for patient screening, treatment, and aftercare can help systematize and standardize the HIFU treatment process. In this fashion, the screening process is linked to the procedure and aftercare. Accurate determination of waist line circumferences is recorded at initiation,[22] and the patient is weighed at every visit and their weight compared to their baseline measurements. Offering counseling on weight maintenance may also be helpful. When patients are held accountable for their weight and BMI, they may be more committed to their treatment.

Before any type of noninvasive treatment, informed consent document is obtained and requisite pre-treatment templates are completed that that record tissue thickness (DUS), the number of zones to be treated, the energy fluence, and the energy deposition mode (e.g. site stack or grid repeat). A simple point and shoot camera may be used to document the treatment zones. Standardized digital photography without underwear is typically utilized to depict pre-treatment and follow-up outcomes. If adverse events occur after treatment, photographic documentation is a necessity.

The patient's waist at the point of greatest abdominal protuberance is measured with a spring-loaded tape at a fixed height off the floor (e.g. measured by laser level). The patient is weighed wearing only a simple tube top and disposable spa-style shorts. Accurate determination of baseline values is essential to ensure comparability to follow-up measurements at 12–16 weeks after treatment. During pre-treatment education patients may be told that it is not uncommon to have some post-treatment ecchymoses.

While the cryolipolysis device is relatively comfortable during treatment, the HIFU fat reduction procedure is somewhat more uncomfortable, given the deeper layer of treatment and the stimulation of superficial sensory nerves deep within the tissue. Discomfort varies with individual pain tolerance and the level of HIFU fluence. A lower fluence level of around 30 J/cm^2 may be better tolerated. Conversely, higher fluence levels are more uncomfortable. Post-treatment dysesthesias and numbness has been reported for up to several weeks after cryolipolysis treatment. Cold appears able to produce structural changes within sensory nerves, although these resolve over time.

Maintaining patient comfort during HIFU should not be challenging, as most individuals with normal pain tolerance can tolerate a treatment without oral sedation. Distracting techniques such as utilizing a vibratory massager on the patient's feet can be helpful. In some cases, oral narcotic pain medicines such as oxycodone or dihydromorphone, anxiolytics, or gabapentin-class medications may be needed for patient comfort.[22] Other sedation approaches include the use of benzodiazopines, oral or parenteral NSAIDs, nitrous oxide, or intravenous agents. Narcotic analgesia exposes patients to the risk of nausea requiring treatment (e.g. with oral disintegrating ondansetron, 4 mg tablet). Directly infiltrated tumescent anesthesia may also be used. Patient comfort during the procedure is better established early in treatment, as it is more difficult to console a patient who is already experiencing procedure-related discomfort.

Patient and operator positioning during the procedure is also important. Use of a softly upholstered massage table with an electric height adjustment may be helpful, as may use of foam blocks and pillows for patient positioning. The treatment provider may similarly be most effective while sitting in an ergonomically designed and comfortable chair. While the Liposonix treatment head/RTC is lightweight and comfortable to hold, attention must be paid to correct ergonomics to avoid repetitive motion fatigue in the operator. Additional patient comfort aids include a warm room (e.g. 22 °C), a blanket or comforter, and slightly dimmed lights. Close attention should be paid to what the patient sees from their perspective on the treatment table – a cluttered room and dirty overhead air vents are potentially anxiety provoking elements. If a vibratory massager is used for patient distraction during the procedure this may require an assistant in addition to the treatment provider. Patient use of headphones and personal music players may impair communication with the treatment provider.

Water is used to couple the Liposonix treatment head to the skin so that the HIFU energy passes from the RTC to the patient. Excessive spraying of water onto the treatment area as a distraction during treatment may contribute to lesser outcomes because of excessive tissue cooling. Additionally, the water pooling may be messy, and the need for containment with towels may become an inconvenience. Ideally, water use should be sufficient to provide for coupling but drenching of the treatment area should be avoided. A dry wash cloth can be used to pick up modest quantities of excess water.

At the completion of treatment, the grid patterns are wiped off the patient and the patient is discharged from the clinic. Patients who have taken oral or parenteral sedation must have someone drive them home. Needless to say, such patients should not operate a vehicle or machinery until their medicated state resolves completely. At discharge, patients are reminded of the possibility of post-treatment ecchymoses that typically resolve after 14 days. They are also told that there may be firmness within the treatment zone for a few weeks.

Changes in body contour after a HIFU treatment start to occur as soon as 4 weeks post-treatment and are complete by 16 weeks.[20] As mentioned earlier, follow-up visits with recording of circumferential standardized measurements and body weight are needed to document clinical outcome and body weight maintenance.

The future of HIFU body contouring looks promising. Future-generation devices may offer custom contouring, based on each individual's laminar anatomy. The current generation device is an excellent starting point for noninvasive body contouring. Physicians can modify fluence levels and other treatment parameters to enable a range of patients to comfortably undergo treatment.

Expected outcomes

HIFU generates high-intensity ultrasound waves that are focused in the deep subcutaneous tissue and cause thermomechanical ablation of SAT as well as collagen remodeling. The safety and efficacy of HIFU has been extensively studied through pre-clinical work and verified in post-marketing trials as well as in a sham-controlled randomized study.

Early work evaluating the utility of HIFU for the treatment of fat reduction was performed in validated porcine models. HIFU energy ranging from 166 to 372 J/cm^2 resulted in a focal target tissue temperature of 70 °C. Gross and microscopic pathology illustrated focal ablation of SAT without damage to surrounding structures, inflammation, or fat necrosis. Additionally, analysis of peripheral blood did not illustrate significant alterations in liver function tests, cholesterol, or free fatty acids.[19]

The safety of HIFU for fat reduction in human subjects was reported by Gadsden and colleagues in 2011.[18] In three clinical trials, 152 healthy men and women with BMI < 30 and with >2.0 cm of SAT in the intended treatment area were treated with HIFU energy doses of 47–331 J/cm^2.[22-24] These subjects included patients undergoing elective abdominoplasty up to 14 weeks after the HIFU treatment. Post-treatment histology and ultrasound revealed well-demarcated disruption of adipocytes within the treatment zone and isolation of HIFU effects limited only to the targeted SAT layer. Additionally, there was no evidence of damage to collateral structures, such as vasculature and nerves. Cellular debris and free fatty acids were phagocytosed at days 14–28, with subsequent hepatic metabolism of free lipids occurring without detectable elevations in serum cholesterol, triglycerides, or free fatty acids. Adverse events were transient and mild, including edema, erythema, dysesthesia, ecchymosis, and discomfort.

The efficacy of HIFU in the treatment of SAT was illustrated in two large series that included 367 patients. In the first report,[25] 282 patients underwent a single HIFU treatment of the anterior abdomen and flanks. Patients had a mean age of 41.3 years and a minimum of 1.5 cm of SAT beyond the planned HIFU focal depth. Histology was studied in a subset of these patients who subsequently underwent elective abdominoplasty after the HIFU treatment. The mean energy dose was 137 J/cm^2, which was divided into two different focal depths and two passes. A mean waist circumference reduction of 4.7 cm was reported 3 months after the single treatment session. Postsurgical abdominoplasty tissue illustrated clearly defined zones of injury that were a consistent and safe distance from the epidermis and dermis. Of note, higher energy levels did not produce larger lesions. Adverse events were mild and transient and included edema, hard lumps, ecchymoses, prolonged tenderness, and pain during treatment. All adverse events resolved in less than 4 weeks except for edema, which resolved in less than 12 weeks. Approximately 13% of treated patients experienced one or more adverse events.

The second series was a retrospective review of 85 patients treated with a single HIFU treatment to the anterior abdomen and flanks. The mean age of subjects was 43.8 years, and a mean energy of 134.8 J/cm^2 with a focal depth of 1.1–1.6 cm resulted in an average circumferential waist reduction of 4.6 cm at 3 months posttreatment. Adverse events were reported by 11.8% of subjects and included prolonged tenderness, ecchymoses, hard lumps, edema, and pain, all of which resolved spontaneously.[26]

Confirmation of the efficacy of HIFU was accomplished through a randomized, single-blind post-market trial[24] as well as a sham-controlled randomized study.[20] Solish et al.[24] evaluated HIFU treatment of the anterior abdomen with subjects randomized to a per-pass fluence group of 47, 52, or 59 J/cm^2, with energy applied in three passes at decreasing depths. The 45 treated patients had mean ages of 42–44 years and mean BMI of 25–27. The vast majority of subjects were Caucasian (79–93%) and female (86–94%). Subject demographics did not differ statistically across treatment groups. Waist circumference was measured in a validated manner at baseline, on the day of treatment, and at follow-up visits at weeks 4, 8, and 12. The primary outcome measure of change in baseline waist circumference at 12 weeks averaged 2.51 cm for all groups. This reduction was a result of treatment of only the abdomen, while other studies previously included flank and abdomen treatment. There was no statistically significant difference in circumference measurements between the three treatment groups at any time point. A majority of patients experienced mild and transient abdominal bruising or redness. There were no serious adverse events.

In a randomized, sham-controlled, single-blinded trial of 180 subjects, treatment with per-pass fluences of 47, 59, or 0 J/cm^2 was applied in three passes to the anterior abdomen and flanks. Treatment resulted in a statistically significant 2.44 cm reduction in the 59 J/cm^2 group at 12 weeks follow-up.[20] The 47 J/cm^2 group did not show a statistically significant reduction in change in baseline waist circumference at 12 weeks. In this study, the average BMI of patients was 25.2, with a mean age of 42.1 years, and the majority were female (85%) and Caucasian (87%). Again, adverse events were transient and mild to moderate, and included edema, ecchymoses, and pain. Additionally, serum lipid and coagulation panels, liver and renal function, and markers of inflammation were not altered with HIFU treatment. In both of the randomized controlled trials, subject weight did not fluctuate substantially from baseline to 12-week follow-up, suggesting that the change seen in waist circumference results derived from HIFU treatment rather than dietary restriction or increased exercise.

Safety

Procedural discomfort

In the randomized, sham-controlled trial, subjects reported greater procedural discomfort at the higher fluence (177 J) compared to the lower fluence (147 J). Discomfort lasted during the procedure and rapidly diminished afterwards.

Ecchymoses

Ecchymoses are the most common adverse event associated with HIFU treatment. Typically, ecchymoses resolve within 14 days.[20]

Tissue firmness

Firmness is the result of inflammation, swelling, and healing after HIFU treatment. Other forms of body contouring, such as conventional or ultrasound-assisted liposuction produce tissue firmness as well. While it may be possible for tissue firmness to represent fat necrosis or masses filled with necrotic oil from tissue heating, this appears to be a very remote adverse event that was not seen in the pivotal trial.

Defined location sensory nerves

HIFU may produce discomfort, which increases with the fluence. Discomfort is particularly marked along known nerve trunks, such as the ilioinguinal nerves, sub-costal nerve pathways, and the chain of sensory nerves that accompany the perforator vessels within the abdominal wall.

Dysesthesias

Dysesthesias may occur after HIFU, but these are self-limited. Gabapentin has been used off-label for the treatment of dysesthesias.

Abnormal laboratory values

These, especially elevated serum lipids, have not been detected. When performed, testing for coagulopathy, liver function, and inflammatory markers has consistently been within normal limits.

Thermal injury to skin

Permanent thermal skin injuries, such as superficial scars, have not been reported.

Deep layer injury

No undesirable or pathologic injuries to deep-layer tissue were detected during the pivotal study. Theoretically, HIFU can induce injuries to deeper tissues, including bone, defined nerve trunks, and muscle. Physicians who offer Liposonix to patients seeking body contouring in areas that have not been approved (i.e. are off-label) are reminded that sub-surface anatomy must be considered, as there are vulnerable motor and sensory nerve trunks that could be affected by HIFU. Examples would be the brachial plexus and upper extremity motor and sensory nerves in the axilla and medial upper arm. Similarly, the sciatic nerve crosses the 'banana roll' area of the sub-gluteal region. The tibial nerve is in the posterior thigh is also potentially within the focal range of the Liposonix HIFU. Finally, the femoral nerve is in the anterior thigh in the vicinity of the inguinal ligament.

Lack of treatment efficacy

Some patients are nonresponders to treatment. Those with thick superficial fat layers, by virtue of their body morphology or BMI >30, may not respond to treatment. Successful outcomes seem to be more common in patients who have just enough MLM for the HIFU to successfully ablate fat and tighten collagen. Patients who cannot maintain their target weight due to weight fluctuations may also not achieve body contour improvement following HIFU. The HIFU treatment is not intended for weight loss.

Repeat treatment

While it is possible to consider repeat treatments with HIFU or even periodic 'maintenance' treatments, there is no data that has been published that studies repeat application of HIFU for fat reduction. It is not known if additional treatments result in greater cumulative fat or circumference reduction.

Tissue effect seen on DUS

It is possible to see extracellular lipid on DUS after a HIFU treatment. This manifests as cloudiness within the treatment zone and is part of the normal biological response whereby ablated adipocytes release lipid. Detectable lipid clears over time with macrophage activity.

Device-related adverse events

The Liposonix device has a variety of sensors which review performance, energy output, and coupling of the device to skin. Safeguard mechanisms will shut down the device if technical faults occur. It is possible for engineers to review the performance parameters of the Liposonix device by accessing the internal computer through the internet.

Operator error

Proper training in the operation of the device is important to minimize the risk of adverse events. Additional operator errors that can affect outcomes pertain to patient selection, how the device is used, and off-label usage. HIFU body contouring is not an 'all-comers' procedure that is appropriate for everyone seeking body contour improvement. Indeed, it is more demanding than some other procedures for the same indications in terms of patient selection and management of expectations. Patient selection with regards to adequate tissue within the treatment area is important, as patients with thin layers of SAT are at risk for HIFU striking deep muscle fascia or bone, both of which are very uncomfortable. Off-label usage of Liposonix in areas such as the inner arms, banana rolls, and posterior thigh has the potential to produce serious adverse events if major nerve trunks are damaged. Outer thighs are safer, as there are no at-risk major nerve trunks in this area.

In summary, the incidence of adverse events when a HIFU treatment is performed by an experienced physician or staff member is very low. Minor, self-limited adverse events are relatively common, and include ecchymoses and transient dysesthesias.

Multi-modality procedures

HIFU can be combined with other modalities to optimize treatment outcomes. While there are no published studies on combination therapies, it is generally believed that complementary technologies may safely be used to enhance patient satisfaction. While HIFU induces collagen remodeling, the primary outcome of HIFU treatment is SAT reduction and not tissue tightening. Thus, additional modalities can be utilized to address tissue laxity. For example, fractional resurfacing, monopolar, hybrid or bipolar radiofrequency, or infrared devices can be coupled with HIFU treatment to achieve both fat reduction and skin tightening.

CASE STUDY 1

A 32-year-old healthy woman presents to your office for potential treatment options for her abdominal contour. She adheres to a healthy diet and exercises 4–5 days per week. Despite her healthy lifestyle, she notes a 'pouch of fat' on her abdomen that is resistant to diet and exercise. She states she is not interested in liposuction as she is apprehensive regarding the recovery process and is interested instead in a procedure that will improve her waistline without any 'surgery'. She is 170 cm in height and weighs 61 kg, with a BMI of 21. She is otherwise healthy, has no chronic medical conditions and takes only a daily multivitamin. On physical examination, she has a localized collection of fat on her anterior abdomen with a pinch test of two finger widths. She has no evidence of umbilical hernia.

This patient would be an ideal candidate for HIFU treatment. She is interested in a noninvasive procedure and has appropriate expectations. Additionally, her BMI is <30, she has a localized area of SAT for treatment, and has no evidence of hernia in the treatment area. Thus, a discussion of the HIFU procedure and projected outcomes is appropriate. Before treatment, a pregnancy test should be performed as this is a contraindication.

CASE STUDY 2

A 48-year-old female patient presents with questions regarding body sculpting. She is particularly interested in treating her abdomen. She is healthy, takes only a daily multivitamin, and had a healthy twin delivery via cesarean section 5 years previously. On physical examination, her abdomen is without evidence of umbilical hernia, a pinch test is one finger breadth in thickness composed of mostly redundant skin and a small amount of subcutaneous fat, and there are numerous striae alba around the umbilicus.

This patient does not have enough subcutaneous adipose tissue in the desired treatment area to undergo HIFU. Her examination is noteworthy for skin laxity as evident by the pinch test and striae, and she does not have a localized collection of subcutaneous adipose tissue of the abdomen. Therefore, a discussion of therapies targeted at skin tightening instead of fat reduction would be appropriate.

References

1. Arnoczky S, Alptek A. Thermal modification of connective tissues: basic science implications and clinical considerations. J Am Acad Orth Surg 2000;8:305–13.
2. Kirn D, Vasconez H, Cibull M, Fink B. Skin contraction with pulsed CO_2 and erbium:YAG laser. Plast Reconstr Surg 1999; 104:2255–60.
3. Seckel B, Younai S, Wang K. Skin tightening effects of the ultrapulse CO_2 laser. Plast Reconstr Surg 1998;102:872–7.
4. Kirsch K, Zelickson BD, Zachary CB, Tope WD. Ultrastructure of collagen thermally denatured by microsecond domain pulsed carbon dioxide laser. Arch Dermatol 1998;134:1255–9.
5. Wall M, Deng XH, Torzilli PA, et al. Thermal modification of collagen. J Shoulder Elbow Surg 1999;8:339–44.
6. Thomsen S. Pathologic analysis of photothermal and photomechanical effects of laser-tissue interactions. Photochem Photobiol 1991;53:825–35.
7. Xu F, Wen T, Lu TJ, Seffen KA. Skin biothermomechanics for medical treatments. J Mech Behav Biomed Materials 2008;1: 172–87.
8. Wright N, Humphrey J. Denaturation of collagen via heating: an irreversible rate process. Annu Rev Biomed Eng 2002;4: 109–28.

9. Dewey W. Arrhenius relationships from the molecule and cell to the clinic. Int J Hyperthermia 1994;10:457–83.

10. Ng E, Chua L. Mesh-independent prediction of skin burns injury. J Mech Eng Tech 2000;24:255–61.

11. Suzuki T, Hirayama T, Aihara K, Hirohata Y. Experimental studies of moderate temperature burns. Burns 1991;17:443–51.

12. Ng E, Chua L. Prediction of skin burn injury: Part 1. Numerical modeling. Proc Inst Mech Eng [H] 2002;216:157–70.

13. Papp A, Kiraly K, Härmä M, et al. The progression of burn depth in experimental burns: a histological and methodological study. Burns 2004;30:684–90.

14. Kister D, Hafemann B, Schmidt K. A model to reproduce predictable full-thickness burns in an experimental animal. Burns Incl Therm Inj 1988;14:297–302.

15. Smahel J. Viability of skin subjected to deep partial thickness thermal damage: experimental studies. Burns 1991;17:17–24.

16. Jiang S, Ma N, Li HJ, Zhang XX. Effect of thermal properties and geometrical dimension on skin burn injury. Burns 2002;28:713–17.

17. Haar GT, Coussios C. High intensity focused ultrasound: physical principles and devices. Int J Hyperthermia 2007;23(2):89–104.

18. Gadsden E, Aguilar MT, Smoller BR, Jewell ML. Evaluation of a novel high-intensity focused ultrasound device for ablating subcutaneous adipose tissue for noninvasive body contouring: safety studies in human volunteers. Aesthet Surg J 2011;31(4):401–10.

19. Jewell ML, Desilets C, Smolle BR. Evaluation of a novel high-intensity focused ultrasound device: preclinical studies in a porcine model. Aesthet Surg J 2011;31(4):429–34.

20. Jewell ML, Baxter RA, Cox SE, et al. Randomized sham-controlled trial to evaluate the safety and effectiveness of a high-intensity focused ultrasound device for noninvasive body sculpting. Plast Reconstr Surg 2011;128(1):253–62.

21. Sasaki GH, Tevez A, Gonzales M. Histological changes after 1440 nm, 1320 nm and 1064 nm wavelength exposures in the deep and superficial layers of human abdominal tissue: acute and delayed findings. White Paper. Westford, MA: Cynosure; 2010.

22. Jewell ML, Weiss RA, Baxter RA, et al. Safety and tolerability of high-intensity focused ultrasonography for noninvasive body sculpting: 24-week data from a randomized, sham-controlled study. Aesthet Surg J 2012;32(7):868–76.

23. Jewell ML, Jewell JL. High intensity focused ultrasound and non-invasive body contouring. In: Rubin J, Jewell ML, Richter DF, Uebel CO, editors. Body contouring and liposuction. Philadelphia: Elsevier; 2013. p. 559–71.

24. Solish N, Lin X, Axford-Gatley RA, et al. A randomized, single-blind, postmarketing study of multiple energy levels of high-intensity focused ultrasound for noninvasive body sculpting. Dermatol Surg 2012;38(1):58–67.

25. Fatemi A. High-intensity focused ultrasound effectively reduces adipose tissue. Semin Cutan Med Surg 2009;28(4):257–62.

26. Fatemi A, Kane MA. High-intensity focused ultrasound effectively reduces waist circumference by ablating adipose tissue from the abdomen and flanks: a retrospective case series. Aesthetic Plast Surg 2010;34(5):577–82.

Liposuction, Ultrasound-assisted and Powered: Fat Reduction

9

Anne Goldsberry, C. William Hanke

Key Messages

- Tumescent liposuction was developed and continues to be widely practiced by dermatologic surgeons
- The tumescent local anesthesia offers significant safety benefits over general anesthesia
- Ultrasonic liposuction may increase the risk of seroma, thermal burns, and necrosis, and consequently should be used with caution
- Powered liposuction, using a reciprocating cannula, increases the rate of fat removal, improves patient recovery, and decreases the physician's physical strain

The history of liposuction

The history of modern liposuction dates to 1976 when Fischer described the use of hollow cannulas to remove subcutaneous fat.[1] Due to the efforts of Fischer, as well as Ilouz and Fournier, cannulas evolved to blunt tipped instruments containing motor driven blades. Ilouz developed the 'wet technique' in which hypotonic saline and hyaluronidase were infiltrated into the subcutaneous tissue prior to suction to achieve anesthesia and mobilize the fat from fibrous attachments.[2,3] In contrast, Fournier introduced the 'criss-cross' technique that allowed for overlapping and intersecting tunnels in the subcutis designed to effect uniform fat reduction.[2,4]

The early liposuction cannulas were 8–10 mm in diameter. With experience, surgeons learned that smaller caliber cannulas were sufficient to remove fat. Smaller cannulas were also beneficial in that they were less likely to damage neurovascular bundles or cause seromas and hematomas. Smaller cannulas allowed for more precise and even contour sculpting, and overall improved aesthetic outcomes. Cannulas today remain small (2–5 mm), with some having an inside diameter of less than 1 mm.[2]

In 1987, Klein introduced the concept of liposuction using 'tumescent technique'.[5] Prior to that time, general anesthesia was required to perform liposuction. Tumescent technique has been refined over time, and is now commonly referred to as tumescent local anesthesia (TLA).[6,7] TLA improved liposuction safety and markedly decreased intraoperative blood loss, thus reducing the overall morbidity associated with liposuction to a negligible level. In the 1980s and early 1990s, numerous American dermatologists adopted TLA and published large studies confirming the superior safety profile of the technique.

Pearl 1

Tumescent anesthesia is a multistage process. Initially, early infiltration provides partial anesthesia which can then be maximized to full tumescence prior to the start of liposuction. Additional 'topping off' of anesthesia may be performed immediately before suctioning or during suctioning, if areas are revealed to have inadequate anesthesia.

The increased adoption of TLA stimulated interest in liposuction and consequently led to the development of adjuvant technologies. In 1988, Zocchi introduced the use of ultrasound-assisted liposuction. Ultrasound-assisted liposuction was met with initial enthusiasm, but unfortunately it was quickly recognized that ultrasound energy delivered into the subcutaneous fat compartment cannot infrequently be associated with complications.[8–10] In the mid-1990s, powered liposuction, using electric reciprocating cannulas, was introduced. Powered liposuction increased the efficiency of tumescent liposuction while maintaining the overall safety of the procedure and hence has been widely adopted.[11]

Patient selection

Liposuction is designed for individuals at or near their ideal body weight who want to reduce single or multiple local accumulations of excess fat. Liposuction is not a weight loss technique. It is important to discuss risks, benefits, and expectations during the initial consultation.

Preoperative evaluation

Performing a thorough preoperative evaluation is essential to maximize the likelihood of patient safety and optimal results. Review of all the patient's medications may reveal medically necessary anticoagulation, which is generally considered a relative contraindication. Medications that thin the blood but are not medically necessary, such a fish oil, nonsteroidal anti-inflammatory drugs, and vitamin E, should be stopped for at least 2 weeks prior to the procedure.[12] Medications that interact with cytochrome P450 3A4 decrease the liver metabolism of lidocaine and consequently could increase toxicity.[13] If possible, these medications should also be stopped at least 2 weeks prior to the liposuction procedure. Preoperative laboratory workup routinely includes complete blood count with differential and platelet count, prothrombin time, partial thromboplastin time, comprehensive chemistry panel, human immunodeficiency virus serology, and hepatitis B and C. An electrocardiogram may be performed for patients over the age of 50.[12]

Once the patient is ready for liposuction, the area to be treated is typically marked and photographed, with specialized symbols used to indicate areas of greater fat accumulation, areas of low fat density to be avoided during liposuction, and areas at the periphery of the target area that are to be lightly suctioned to avoid an abrupt step-off shelf, or 'feathered.' The patient is then prepped under sterile conditions and the remainder of the procedure is performed clean or sterile. Oral anxiolysis such as medium-duration benzodiazepines (e.g. diazepam) may not only help the patient better cope emotionally with the mild procedure-associated discomfort but also directly relax abdominal and other musculature to facilitate lidocaine infiltration and suctioning.

Anesthesia

TLA is based on a lidocaine solution in which normal saline is used as the diluent. Sodium bicarbonate 8.4% is added to buffer the solution, with 10 mL of sodium bicarbonate 8.4% usually mixed in per 1000 mL of normal saline. In order to induce vasoconstriction, which facilitates hemostasis and decreases the rate of absorption of the lidocaine, 1 mL of epinephrine 1:1000 is added per 1000 mL of normal saline. The concentration of lidocaine in TLA is normally between 0.05% and 0.1%. New studies have demonstrated adequate anesthesia with lidocaine concentrations as low as 0.04–0.05%,[13] but more sensitive sites with greater sensory innervations may require slightly higher concentrations. The total volume of tumescent solution is usually kept at a level not exceeding 55 mg/kg, which is a dose level that is known to be safe.[14]

Entry sites are prepared by intradermal infiltration using full strength lidocaine solution, such as 1% lidocaine with 1:100000 epinephrine. Incisions for cannula entry sites are typically made with a No. 11 blade or a 2 mm punch biopsy device. A blunt tipped infiltration cannula or a medium diameter needle (e.g. 18–22 gauge) is inserted, and the TLA solution is delivered into the subcutaneous space using an infiltration pump. After approximately 20–60 minutes, the epinephrine should reach maximum vasoconstrictive effect with maximal intercellular diffusion.

Operative technique

The suction cannula is inserted vertically, redirected to the horizontal plane, and then repositioned so that the cannula aperture is facing downwards, away from the overlying dermis. Tunneling with the cannula is conducted using meticulous, linear strokes, in a fan-like pattern radiating circumferentially from the incision point. Long strokes that comprise almost the entire length of the cannula should be used so that fat is removed consistently and evenly, and small areas are not oversuctioned so as to create indentations. The nondominant hand, or 'smart hand', may be placed on the skin overlying the cannula tip to monitor the cannula position. The use of multiple entry sites facilitates a criss-cross pattern to optimize contour. Suction should be parallel to the axis of lymphatic drainage to minimize tissue trauma. To stabilize the tissue, use of MASST, manually assisted skin stabilization technique, is helpful. In this technique, an assistant stretches the skin providing traction on the skin surface.[12] Operating technique varies according to surgeon and anatomic region.

Liposuction of the neck and jowls is an effective treatment to remove submental fat, which is often hereditary. Initial markings may identify key anatomic structures, so that liposuction can be appropriately targeted and danger zones, such as the point at which the marginal mandibular nerve courses over the mandibular rim, can be avoided. Patients can be positioned supine with the head extended. TLA commences with infiltration of a small (100–150 mL) volume of anesthesia to establish numbness. Further infiltration is then typically continued until tumescence is achieved, and, in some cases, additional infiltration, so-called 'topping off', may be used to add yet more tumescence before suction begins. Short cannulas with a diameter of 1.5–3 mm are commonly used.

The abdomen is the most common site of body liposuction. It is important to identify which areas within the abdomen require suction. Individuals with focal excess adiposity in the lower abdomen respond well to isolated suction of the lower abdomen. However, isolated lower abdominal suction in patients with more diffuse fatty deposition can result in an overhanging upper abdomen, and so typically both lower and upper abdomens are suctioned concurrently. Suction may continue to the lateral flank area to avoid an abrupt step-off. Patients are positioned supine (Fig. 9.1) before the procedure begins. Typically five or six entry sites are used, but more may be required. Suction should include the mid-fat and also target deeper fat planes to ensure adequate fat removal while avoiding surface dimpling. Meticulous anesthesia and suctioning around the umbilicus is needed to avoid residual excess fat at this location, and hence a protuberant umbilical area postoperatively.

Liposuction of the hips, thighs and buttock requires careful evaluation of the musculature and skin quality on the lower extremities. For the thighs and hips, patients are routinely positioned in the lateral decubitus position (Figs 9.2–9.4). For the buttock, patients tend to be positioned prone. Care should be taken to remove equal amounts of fat from both sides. Oversuctioning will result in an unnatural concave contour.

Liposuction of the arms is used to treat excess fatty deposits. It is most commonly performed on the upper arms, but can occasionally extend to the forearms and shoulders. Patients are typically supine, and the arm is repositioned as necessary throughout the procedure (Fig. 9.5). Excessive suctioning of the arms can worsen their appearance, with fatty arms replaced by arms with excess skin; this possibility is typically discussed with patients before surgery, and it may be prudent to apprise patients that further skin excision may be appropriate after liposuction.

Liposuction of the male breast is indicated for treatment of pseudogynecomastia, or increased fat accumulation in the male breast. A preoperative mammogram is

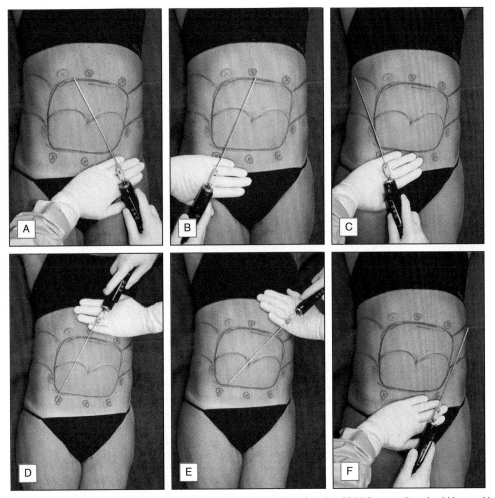

Figure 9.1 (A–F) During liposuction of the abdomen, the patient should be positioned supine. Multiple entry sites should be used in both the upper and lower abdomen. Suction should be formed in a fan-like pattern targeting deeper fat planes. Lateral entry sites can be used to access the flanks *(courtesy of C. William Hanke)*

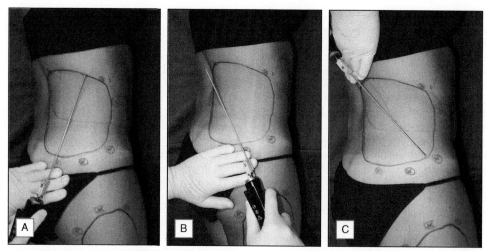

Figure 9.2 (A–C) Liposuction of the hips is performed with the patient in the lateral decubitus position *(courtesy of C. William Hanke)*

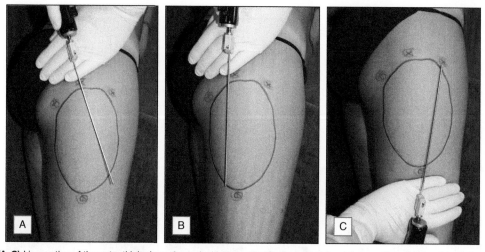

Figure 9.3 (A–C) Liposuction of the outer thighs is performed with the patient in the lateral decubitus position. Entry points at the upper thigh and mid-thigh are used to keep the cannula parallel to the long axis of the body *(courtesy of C. William Hanke)*

sometimes necessary to rule out gynecomastia, or enlargement of the mammary gland. Because the breast is very sensitive, TLA should be performed slowly using small caliber cannulas or needles, and a relatively high concentration of tumescent anesthesia may be preferable. Using three or four incisions in an arc in the inframammary fold optimizes the criss-cross technique while successfully concealing the minimal scars that are thus created. The goal should be to suction as much fat as possible.

Liposuction of the female breast has emerged as an alternative to surgical breast reduction for women who are willing to accept a 30–50% breast volume reduction.[15,16] The patient is usually positioned supine with the ipsilateral arm behind the head. Three to four incisions are made in the inframammary crease. Suction typically commences in the deeper planes and gradually moves to the superficial fat. As usual, suction is usually performed in a fan-like pattern. Very high levels of patient satisfaction have been

reported, but it should be noted that preoperative malposition or ptosis of the nipple–areolar complex cannot be rectified by liposuction alone.[15]

Endpoints include time spent suctioning a given area, the volume of fat suctioned, patient discomfort, increasing amounts of blood in the aspirate, and physical assessment of the area by palpation. Once liposuction is mostly completed, the patient may be gradually moved to a sitting or standing position, with appropriate support, to assess bilateral symmetry and to correct any remaining pockets of fat. In general, no more than 5 L of fat should be suctioned in a single session so as to avoid excess intravascular fluid shifts and the risk of seroma.

Complications

All patients should expect to have some degree of bruising, swelling, soreness, redness of the incision sites and

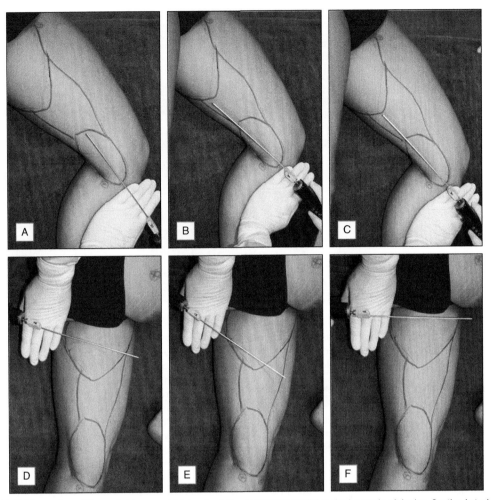

Figure 9.4 (A–F) Liposuction of the medial knee and thighs should be performed parallel to the long axis of the leg. Suction is typically performed starting at the medial knee, moving up through a transition zone in the medial mid-thigh, and ending with the medial upper thigh. Suction of the transition zone is essential to maintain normal contour of the medial thighs. Of note, the upper medial thigh is the only location where liposuction is performed perpendicular to the long axis of the body in a criss-cross fashion *(courtesy of C. William Hanke)*

fatigue in the days following the procedure. Fatigue usually remits within 1–2 days, and the other normal sequelae resolve within 1–2 weeks. Infrequent complications include bleeding, hematoma, seroma, infection, and lidocaine toxicity. To date, there has never been a fatality with liposuction using tumescent local anesthesia when appropriate guidelines are followed. Surface irregularities or persistent edema improve with time. Patients may be counseled not to judge the result until 6 months or more postoperatively. Further interventions and touch-ups are often delayed for 1 year or more postoperatively.

Safety studies

The safety of liposuction using TLA has been supported by a number of large studies. In 1988, Bernstein and Hanke published a multicenter retrospective review of 9478 liposuction cases performed by dermatologic sur-

geons.[17] There were no significant complications. In 1995, Hanke and colleagues reviewed 15 336 patients who underwent tumescent liposuction in 44 014 body areas performed by dermatologic surgeons. There were no major complications such as death, embolism, hypovolemic shock, perforation of peritoneum or thorax, thrombophlebitis or blood loss requiring transfusion.[18] In 2002, Housman and colleagues reviewed 66 570 liposuction cases performed by dermatologic surgeons.[19] Again there were no fatalities. A total of 35 (0.0015%) major adverse events were reported.

In contrast, the plastic surgery literature shows higher rates of complications. In 2000, a survey of plastic surgeons performing 496 245 liposuction cases under general anesthesia showed a fatality rate of 19.1/100 000.[20] The causes of the fatalities included thromboembolism (23.1%), abdomen/visceral perforation (14.6%), anesthesia/sedation/medication (10%), fat embolism

Figure 9.5 (A, B) Liposuction of the posterior upper arm (i.e. triceps area) should be performed with the cannula parallel to the long axis of the arm. The arm is often repositioned several times during the procedure *(courtesy of C. William Hanke)*

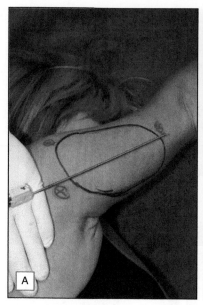 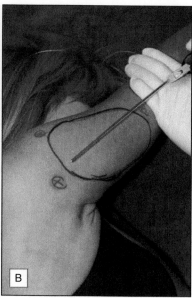

(8.5%), cardiorespiratory failure (5.4%), massive infection (5.4%), and hemorrhage (4.6%).[20] In over a quarter of patients, the cause of death could not be determined.[20]

Ultrasound-assisted liposuction

Ultrasonic energy used in conjunction with liposuction was first presented by Zocchi at the Congress of French Society of Aesthetic Surgery in Paris in 1988.[8–10] He subsequently published a series of 280 patients treated with ultrasonic liposculpture. Zocchi suggested that the use of ultrasonic energy delivered through titanium probes allowed for more efficient removal of adipocytes as the ultrasonic energy resulted in a 'lifting of the treated areas' in comparison to liposuction alone.[21]

Ultrasound used in conjunction with liposuction converts electrical energy to rapid ultrasonic vibrations via a piezoelectric crystal, with this mechanical energy then dissipated as heat within the tissue. Ultrasonic energy is delivered internally, via insertion of a solid metal rod or hollow metal cannula. The resulting thermal energy preferentially liquefies the low density subcutaneous fat tissue while sparing the higher density connective tissue and neurovascular bundles. This facilitates selective removal of the fat.[8–10]

Pearl 5

Careful and complete tumescent infiltration with needles or infiltration cannulae followed by a waiting period of 20–60 minutes is needed to avoid inadequately treated 'hot spots' that are tender and hence an obstacle to subsequent suctioning.

Use of ultrasound-assisted liposuction has been controversial. Advocates argue that ultrasound decreases bleed-ing as a result of selective liquefaction of the fat and decreases damage to connective tissue and neurovascular structures. Critics assert that the decreased blood can be attributed to the tumescent anesthesia that is required to perform the procedure.[10] Supporters also argue that the technology reduces surgeon strain, therefore conserving energy for more precise body contouring.[8]

The majority of the criticism results from the increased complication rates associated with the technology. Much of the literature addressing ultrasound-assisted liposuction has been anecdotal, with many surgeons abandoning the technology prior to the availability of any controlled studies. In 1998, Maxwell and Gingrass, who reviewed 250 of their own cases, reported that ultrasound-assisted liposuction was 'safe and effective'. They did note three cases of dermal necrosis (1.2%), 28 postoperative seromas (11.2%), and 35 Reston foam blisters (14%). Of note, the authors attributed Reston foam blisters to the postoperative dressing, and concluded that they were unrelated to the use of ultrasound.[8] Klein notes that seromas occur in approximately 15–70% of patients treated with ultrasound-assisted liposuction.[22] Burns and skin necrosis have been reported in approximately 4%.[23]

The increased number of complications associated with ultrasound is believed to be the result of mild to moderate temperature elevations of the skin. Increased temperature appears to lead to a procoagulant state, and subsequent microvascular thrombosis and tissue damage. In an evaluation of tissue temperatures during ultrasound-assisted liposuction, Ablaza and colleagues noted that one of 55 patients in the study had a subcutaneous temperature elevation to 41 °C during the procedure.[24] Although the temperature elevation was only noted in an individual patient, the potential consequences are very significant if such elevations are routine.

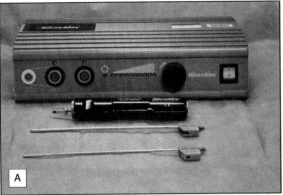

Figure 9.6 (A) MicroAire® powered liposuction device and cannulae. **(B)** Handpiece with attached cannula *(with permission, MicroAire Surgical Instruments, Inc., Charlottesville, VA)*

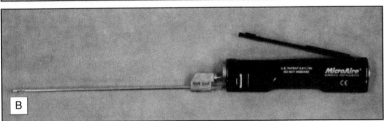

In the authors' opinion, the increased incidence of complications from ultrasound-assisted liposuction outweigh any potential benefits of the procedure.

Powered liposuction

Powered liposuction was developed in the mid to late 1990s. Like ultrasound-assisted liposuction, it was designed to facilitate ease of movement of the cannula through the subcutaneous tissue, but powered liposuction was intended to avoid thermal complications of the type associated with ultrasonic energy. Powered liposuction cannulas evolved from early versions with external blades to those with internal blades and finally to vibrating cannulas. The cannulas move several millimeters in a reciprocating, or to and fro, motion at a rate of 800–10 000 movements per minute.[11]

Pearl 6

Powered liposuction is helpful in all body areas, especially fibrous areas such as the male breast.

The initial powered liposuction equipment required compressed gas. The equipment was noisy, and storage of the large gas tanks was problematic.[11]

Electric-powered liposuction equipment was the next advance. Wells Johnson (Tucson, Arizona) developed the Rojas reciprocating cannula. The unit had a 12 ounce handpiece, 3 mm stroke distance, and moved at 26 000 vibrations per minute. Sattler introduced the VibraSat (Moller Medical, Germany) device. The handpiece is heavy at over 24 ounces, has a 2.8 mm stroke distance, and has an adjustable vibration rate. The Byron ACR reciprocating cannula (Byron Medical, Tucson, Arizona) has a disposable handpiece, 12.7 mm stroke distance, and vibrates at 0–800 per minute. This device is noisy and has the recurring cost of disposable handles. Finally, MicroAire's PAL® (MicroAire Surgical Instruments Inc., Charlottesville, VA) has been the most widely adopted powered suction device (Fig. 9.6). It has a 19.2 ounce handpiece with a 2 mm stroke distance. The cannula vibrates at 24 000–240 000 strokes per minute. Advantages include lower noise and increased precision, but the handpiece is heavy. On average, electric-powered liposuction equipment costs are $5000–$13 000.[11,25]

Powered liposuction has been found to have a number of benefits over traditional liposuction.[26] Katz and co-workers performed a paired comparison study of 21 patients who underwent powered liposuction on one side of the body and traditional liposuction on the contralateral side. Powered liposuction resulted in a 35% shorter procedure time, 31% greater fat aspiration per minute, 45% less intraoperative pain, and 49% reduction in surgeon strain. The study also highlighted postoperative advantages including a 38% reduction in postoperative pain, a 37% reduction in ecchymoses, a 32% reduction in edema, and overall faster recovery.[11]

Similarly, Coleman et al.[27] evaluated the efficacy of powered liposuction in a study of four powered liposuction devices, each with both the powered mode on and powered mode off. The rate of fat extraction increased by 20–45% when the powered devices were turned on. Following the procedures, 54% of patients said they preferred powered liposuction and 46% had no preference;

none preferred traditional liposuction. Patients reported a 'comforting' feeling with the powered liposuction.[27]

Coleman and colleagues also evaluated the learning curve associated with transitioning from traditional liposuction to powered liposuction equipment. Surgeons who had performed seven or fewer powered liposuction cases experienced a 2% decrease in the rate of fat extraction when turning on the powered suction. In contrast, surgeons that had performed eight or more powered liposuction cases experienced a 45% increase in the rate of fat extraction when turning on the powered suction.[27]

Despite initial concerns that the movement of the cannula would increase the potential for seroma formation, powered liposuction has been found to have a similar safety profile to traditional nonpowered liposuction using tumescent anesthesia. In a series of 207 cases of powered liposuction performed by a dermatologic surgeon and a plastic surgeon, Katz et al. noted seroma development in 1.4% of patients, but no significant associated complications.[28] Similarly, Coleman and colleagues evaluated 50 powered liposuction patients and noted no significant increase in complications compared with traditional liposuction.[27]

Pearl 7

Liposuction endpoints include time spent suctioning a given area, the volume of fat suctioned, patient discomfort, increasing amounts of blood in the aspirate, and physical assessment of the treatment area by palpation.

CASE STUDY 1
Powered liposuction for pseudogynecomastia

A 21-year-old man was overweight as a child and teenager. He weighed 215 pounds at the age of 16 years, then lost 70 pounds following a diet and exercise program. At age 21, the patient was 70 inches tall and weighed 165 pounds. He complained about large breasts that had not resolved with the weight loss program. Physical examination revealed a normal 21-year-old man with symmetric enlargement of both breasts. A diagnosis of pseudogynecomastia was made.

The patient underwent liposuction of both breasts using TLA:

- A total TLA volume of 1700 mL containing 0.1% lidocaine and 1 : 1 000 000 epinephrine was administered using a 1.5 inch 20-gauge needle and a Klein pump

- 800 mL of fat and fluid were aspirated using a MicroAire powered 4 mm diameter reciprocating cannula.

The aspiration was performed through four small incisions in the inframammary fold of each breast. The patient tolerated the procedure well and healed uneventfully. Pre- and postoperative photographs reveal marked flattening of both breasts with a normal appearance (Fig. 9.7).

CASE STUDY 2
Powered liposuction for lipedema

A 50-year-old woman was referred by an endocrinologist for evaluation of lipedema. Accumulation of unsightly subcutaneous fat had developed progressively for 5 years on the lower half of the body. Continuous aching pain in the legs prevented the patient from exercising comfortably.

The patient's weight at the time of examination was 155 pounds; she had weighed 180 pounds 5 years previously. The body areas above the waist were normal on examination. Dysmorphic subcutaneous fat accumulations were present on the outer and inner thighs, hips, inner knees, and legs.

Liposuction of the outer and inner thighs was performed using TLA:

- 4.5 L of TLA solution containing 0.05–0.075% lidocaine with 1 : 1 000 000 epinephrine was delivered to the treatment areas using a 20-gauge 1.5 inch needle and a Klein pump
- The areas were aspirated using a MicroAire powered 4.0 mm diameter cannula

- 2325 mL of fluid was aspirated including 1650 mL of yellow fat. The patient tolerated the procedure well and recovered routinely.

The patient was able to exercise without leg pain within 4 weeks following the procedure. The patient's body weight decreased to 141 pounds after several months.

Liposuction of the inner knees and upper legs was performed 8 months later:

- 1100 mL TLA solution was utilized
- 500 mL fluid including 350 mL yellow fat was aspirated using powered liposuction as previously described.

The patient continues her pain-free exercise regimen to the present and has maintained her body weight at 140 pounds. Pre- and postoperative photographs reveal contour improvement in all of the treated areas (Fig. 9.8).

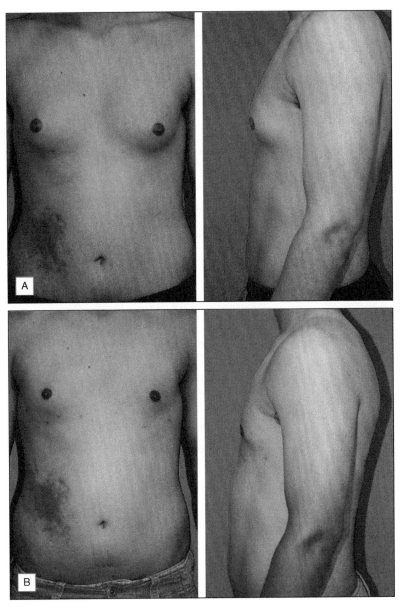

Figure 9.7 (A) A 21-year-old man has pseudogynecomastia involving both breasts. **(B)** The breasts are much flatter and appear normal 6 months after powered liposuction using TLA *(courtesy of C. William Hanke)*

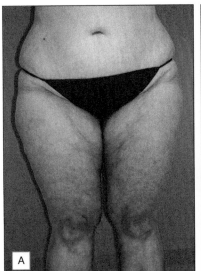
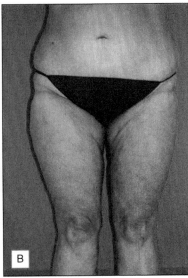

Figure 9.8 (A) A 50-year-old woman has lipedema involving the inner and outer thighs, inner knees, and legs. The patient cannot exercise due to continuous pain in the legs. **(B)** The inner and outer thighs, inner knees, and upper legs demonstrate contour improvement following two powered liposuction procedures using TLA. The patient was able to exercise without leg pain following the liposuction procedure *(courtesy of C. William Hanke)*

References

1. Fischer G. Liposculpture: the 'correct' history of liposuction. Part I. J Dermatol Surg Oncol 1990;16(12):1087–9.

2. Flynn TC, Coleman WP 2nd, Field LM, et al. History of liposuction. Dermatol Surg 2000;26(6):515–20.

3. Illouz YG. Body contouring by lipolysis: a 5-year experience with over 3000 cases. Plast Reconstr Surg 1983;72(5):591–7.

4. Fournier P. Body sculpting through syringe liposuction and autologous fat re-injection. Corona del Mar: Samuel Rolf International; 1987.

5. Klein JA. The tumescent technique for liposuction surgery. Am J Cosmet Surg 1987;4:263–7.

6. Sommer B, Sattler G, Hanke CW. Tumeszenz-Lokalanasthesie. Berlin: Springer; 1999.

7. Hanke CW, Sommer D, Sattler G. Tumescent local anesthesia. Berlin: Springer; 2001.

8. Maxwell GP, Gingrass MK. Ultrasound-assisted lipoplasty: a clinical study of 250 consecutive patients. Plast Reconstr Surg 1998;101(1):189–202, discussion 3–4.

9. Kenkel JM, Robinson JB Jr, Beran SJ, et al. The tissue effects of ultrasound-assisted lipoplasty. Plast Reconstr Surg 1998; 102(1):213–20.

10. Klein JA. Critique of ultrasonic liposuction. In: Klein JA, editor. Tumescent technique, tumescent anesthesia and microcannular liposuction. St Louis: Mosby; 2000.

11. Katz BE, Maiwald DC. Power liposuction. Dermatol Clin 2005;23(3):383–91, v.

12. Hanke CW, Sattler S, Sommer B. Textbook of liposuction. Abingdon: Informa Healthcare; 2007.

13. Habbema L. Efficacy of tumescent local anesthesia with variable lidocaine concentration in 3430 consecutive cases of liposuction. J Am Acad Dermatol 2010;62(6):988–94.

14. Ostad A, Kageyama N, Moy RL. Tumescent anesthesia with a lidocaine dose of 55 mg/kg is safe for liposuction. Dermatol Surg 1996;22(11):921–7.

15. Habbema L. Breast reduction using liposuction with tumescent local anesthesia and powered cannulas. Dermatol Surg 2009; 35(1):41–52, discussion 52.

16. Matarasso A, Courtiss EH. Suction mammaplasty: the use of suction lipectomy to reduce large breasts. Plast Reconstr Surg 1991;87(4):709–17.

17. Bernstein G, Hanke CW. Safety of liposuction: a review of 9478 cases performed by dermatologists. J Dermatol Surg Oncol 1988;14(10):1112–14.

18. Hanke CW, Bernstein G, Bullock S. Safety of tumescent liposuction in 15 336 patients. National survey results. Dermatol Surg 1995;21(5):459–62.

19. Housman TS, Lawrence N, Mellen BG, et al. The safety of liposuction: results of a national survey. Dermatol Surg 2002;28(11):971–8.

20. Grazer FM, de Jong RH. Fatal outcomes from liposuction: census survey of cosmetic surgeons. Plast Reconstr Surg 2000;105(1):436–46, discussion 447–8.

21. Zocchi ML. Ultrasonic assisted lipoplasty. Technical refinements and clinical evaluations. Clin Plast Surg 1996;23(4):575–98.

22. Klein JA. Critique of ultrasonic liposuction. In: Klein JA, editor. Tumescent technique, tumescent anesthesia and microcannular liposuction. St Louis: Mosby; 2000.

23. Schelflan M, Tazi H. Ultrasonic-assisted body contouring. Aesthet Surg J 1996;16:197.

24. Ablaza VJ, Gingrass MK, Perry LC, et al. Tissue temperatures during ultrasound-assisted lipoplasty. Plast Reconstr Surg 1998; 102(2):534–42.

25. Geiger JM, Frew KE, Katz BE. Powered liposuction: results and complications. In: Hanke CW, Sattler G, editors. Liposuction. Procedures in Cosmetic Dermatology. Philadelphia: Saunders; 2005.

26. Katz BE, Bruck MC, Coleman WP 3rd. The benefits of powered liposuction versus traditional liposuction: a paired comparison analysis. Dermatol Surg 2001;27(10):863–7.

27. Coleman WP 3rd, Katz B, Bruck M, et al. The efficacy of powered liposuction. Dermatol Surg 2001;27(8):735–8.

28. Katz BE, Bruck MC, Felsenfeld L, Frew KE. Power liposuction: a report on complications. Dermatol Surg 2003;29(9):925–7, discussion 927.

Laser Lipolysis: Fat Reduction

Anthony M. Rossi, Kira Minkis, Murad Alam,
Michael S. Kaminer, Bruce E. Katz

10

Key Messages

- Laser-assisted lipolysis is an effective procedure for localized adipose removal that may also induce simultaneous skin tightening
- The mechanism of action of laser-assisted lipolysis includes photo-acoustic, photomechanical, and photothermal effects
- Fibrous areas, previously treated areas, and areas of fat accumulation that have overlying skin laxity are some examples of areas amenable to laser-assisted liposuction

Introduction

Since its inception, lipoplasty, or liposuction, has continued to evolve with the addition of ultrasound-assisted, power-assisted, and then laser-assisted liposuction.

Since its approval by the Food and Drug Administration (FDA) in 2006, laser-assisted lipolysis (LAL) has become an integral tool used by many surgeons for simultaneous adipose removal and tissue tightening in selected patients. According to the Cosmetic Surgery National Data Bank, in 2010 liposuction of all types was the second most common cosmetic surgical procedure, with an estimated 289016 cases, an increase of 63.4% from 1997.[1] Liposuction was the most common cosmetic surgical procedure performed in men in 2010, and it was also the most common surgical procedure in the 35- to 50-year-old age category.

The evolution of liposuction has mirrored the desire to improve upon the standard. In the context of patient demand for improved results, shorter downtime, and fewer adverse events, LAL offers flexibility, in that the laser can be utilized solely to destroy adipocytes or can be used in combination with more traditional liposuction techniques. While true LAL is indeed an invasive procedure, the use of the laser alone or as an adjuvant to traditional liposuction has been purported to reduce blood loss due to coagulation of blood vessels, faster healing time, and less patient downtime.[2]

Evolution and mechanism of action

The laser–tissue interaction occurring in LAL is based on the well-established mechanism of selective photothermolysis, described by Anderson et al.[3]; here the chromophores are adipose tissue and water.

Pearl 1

Chromophores targeted in laser-assisted liposuction include adipose tissue and water

Apfelberg[4] was the first to conduct trials utilizing LAL. Initial experiments were with a 40 W, 0.2 second pulse duration, 600 μm diameter Nd:YAG fiber that was housed in a 4–6 mm cannula. The fiber was not in direct contact with the fatty tissue and early findings suggested that this technique decreased patient pain, edema, postoperative bruising, and edema.[4] A pulsed, 1064 nm Nd:YAG laser transmitted by an optical fiber, housed within a 1 mm cannula, which came into direct contact with adipose tissue, was then tried. It was reported that adipocyte lysis resulted directly from the laser energy. It was also concluded that the procedure had other beneficial effects compared with traditional liposuction, as further demonstrated by Badin and colleagues, who showed LAL decreased intraoperative blood loss and postoperative ecchymoses, and improved skin tightening.[5] Of clinical significance was the observation that LAL was associated with stimulation of neocollagenesis in the dermal layer and dermal–adipose interface. This was believed to account for the purported cutaneous tightening and improved skin redraping seen postoperatively. Ichikawa and colleagues found that adipose cells directly treated with a 1064 nm Nd:YAG laser demonstrated greater histologic evidence of injury than nonlaser-irradiated adipose tissue that had been suctioned, and that laser treatment was associated with dose-dependent adipose lysis, and collagen fiber coagulation.[6]

So as to improve results associated with LAL and to prevent collateral thermal damage, multiple wavelengths have been employed based on their preferential absorption by adipose and water compared with 1064 nm (Table 10.1). Compared with a 1064 nm wavelength, a 1440 nm

Table 10.1 Multiple wavelengths employed based on absorption by adipose and water

Wavelength	Adipose	Water
1064 nm	1	1
924 nm	2.8	1.4
980 nm	1.7	3.6
1320 nm	5.9	11.5
1440 nm	127	252

wavelength demonstrates greater fat absorption with less tissue penetration and scatter. This may be warranted in certain delicate areas where collateral thermal damage can lead to a higher risk of scarring.

Mordon et al.[7] utilized a continuous-wave 980 nm diode laser (Pharaon®, Osyris, Hellemmes, France) to target adipose. Evidence of carbonization within the adipose tissue and collagen fibers was detected, which was thought to be due to a combination of the higher laser fluence and continuous waveform.[7] It may be therefore deduced that a pulsed wave laser with shorter pulse duration would allow for the thermal relaxation of the target chromophore and therefore less collateral thermal destruction.

The preferential absorption of laser energy by adipocytes causes deformation of the adipocyte and volume expansion leading to cell lysis. The adipocytes that are closest to the laser fiber tip are exposed to the highest fluence and undergo photo-acoustic/photomechanical destruction. Surrounding adipocytes are exposed to lesser fluences and are therefore subject to more photothermal-based damage. This may result in cellular changes but not necessarily immediate cell lysis. The immediately destroyed adipocytes as well as the thermally injured cells, which may eventually lyse, are the damaged adipocytes which are theorized to be undergoing apoptosis and eventual removal by phagocytosis, possibly via activated macrophages.[8]

Additionally, salutary effects of LAL such as decreased postoperative blood loss may be due to the absorption of energy by oxyhemoglobin and methemoglobin. The 1064 nm device has absorption peaks for both chromophores, with methemoglobin being preferred, possibly accounting for the coagulation effects seen. The theorized associated end benefit of LAL is the effect on skin tightening and redraping. This is thought to be due to a photo-stimulatory effect due to the collateral thermal energy acting upon dermal and adipose collagen. Lower energy levels farther away from the laser tip are sufficient to cause thermal heating but not complete destruction of collagen.[9]

The photothermal effects of LAL, like those of any laser procedure, must not be underestimated. Bulk heating in any one location can produce deleterious effects. This can include thermal burns and cutaneous necrosis. Empiri-

cal findings suggest that an internal temperature between 48 °C and 50 °C must be reached for collagen denaturation and subsequent skin tightening, and therefore many new devices are being equipped with an internal temperature gauge to cease laser firing if the temperature at the fiber tip exceeds a corresponding threshold. External temperatures between 38 °C and 41 °C have been identified as safe and efficacious.[10] This skin surface temperature can also be monitored with the use of an external infrared thermal probe.

Patient selection

With any elective cosmetic procedure, patient selection and patient education are key components to a successful outcome. Patient selection and consultation start as soon as a patient expresses interest in the procedure. Patients may vary in their degree of knowledge of 'laser lipolysis'. Some patients may expect an external laser device, and not an invasive procedure, so it is important to understand the base knowledge and expectations of each patient. The educational process can be initiated when a patient calls the office inquiring about the procedure or, via a patient questionnaire when a patient presents for the initial consultation. The more informed and realistic the patient expectations, the more 'successful' the procedure will be.

Indications

LAL is indicated for the localized destruction of adipose tissue as well as skin tightening, with the latter effect distinguishing it from traditional liposuction. Areas in which LAL has been used effectively include the abdomen (Figs 10.1 and 10.2), flanks (Fig. 10.1), upper arms (Fig. 10.3), submental/neck area (Fig. 10.4), back, inner and outer thighs, knees, calves, and ankles. LAL may also be suitable for patients who have had previous procedures such as traditional liposuction.

> **Pearl 2**
>
> Laser lipolysis with or without subsequent aspiration of fat can be useful for areas of recalcitrant adiposity remaining after previous procedures.

Fibrous adipose tissue areas are commonly encountered in areas such as the male breast, hips, and particularly the back. Due to the fibrous elements at these sites, these areas may be responsive to LAL, which can release fat encased fibrous tissue with decreased trauma. Also, since a relatively smaller cannula size can be used during LAL, trauma may be mitigated compared with the use of larger cannula sizes typically needed for traditional liposuction. LAL has also been used to remove lipomas.[11]

Patient evaluation

As with traditional liposuction, real time patient evaluation and examination are crucial to understanding patient

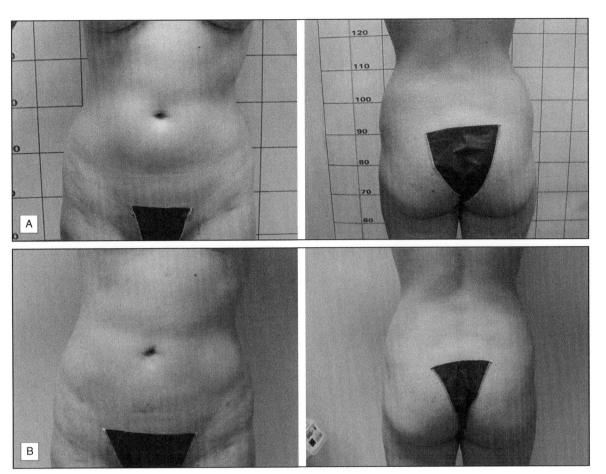

Figure 10.1 (A) Before and **(B)** 3 months after laser-assisted lipolysis to the abdomen (left) and flanks (right). Note bilateral lower abdomen entry points done with 1.5 mm punch biopsy tool and left to heal by secondary intention

concerns and expectations prior to LAL. Realistic expectations regarding the timeline of events, postoperative care required, degree of fat removal, and degree of tissue tightening can also be conveyed at this juncture. Patients may physically highlight their areas of concern, as their linguistic representations may be inaccurate. For instance, when a patient refers to the 'flank area', he or she may in fact be thinking of a different anatomical location. Patients may also be made aware of fat pockets in contiguous regions that may require additional treatment to achieve the best overall results; for example, focal LAL of the lower abdomen may leave a patient with a full, overhanging, upper abdomen.

> ### Pearl 3
>
> Topics that should emphasized during the consultation in addition to routine preoperative screening include postoperative care and bruising, degree of fat removal, time to see full results (3–6 months), and realistic expectations of skin tightening.

Preoperatively, a thorough medical, surgical, medication, and allergy history should be obtained. Over-the-counter and herbal medications should also be considered. Many of these medications can interact with the metabolization of tumescent anesthesia through activation or inhibition of cytochrome P450 enzymes. Medications that are contraindicated include warfarin, clopidogrel bisulfate, aspirin, nonsteroidal anti-inflammatory drugs, and other anticoagulants, as these will increase the risk of bleeding and hematoma formation. Pregnancy or lactation are also contraindications.

The ideal candidate would be someone who is in good health, maintains a healthy diet, enjoys stable weight, and exercises regularly. In the context of LAL, a healthy patient is generally an American Society of Anesthesiologists' Physical Status Classification System class I or II, that is, either 'normal healthy patient', or 'mild system disease and no functional limitation', respectively. Requesting medical clearance may be appropriate for patients over 60 years of age and those who have a history of cardiovascular disease, hypertension, or diabetes.

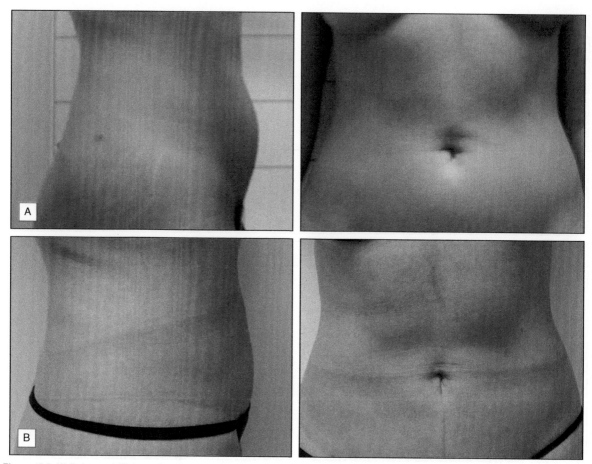

Figure 10.2 (A) Before and **(B)** 3 months after laser-assisted lipolysis to the abdomen, side view (left) and frontal view (right)

Patient evaluation checklist

- Past medical history: highlight clotting or bleeding disorders, liver disease
- Past surgical history – related to the area being treated, including pre-existing scars
- Medication use/drug allergies
- Physical exam: standing position
- Diet history
- Baseline body weights
- Circumference of area of interest
- Body mass index (BMI)
- Baseline images
- Consent forms
- Baseline blood laboratories: complete metabolic profile, complete blood count with platelet count, liver function tests, prothrombin and partial thromboplastin time, hepatitis B/C serologies, human immunodeficiency virus serologies, beta-human chorionic gonadotropin pre-surgery/urine pregnancy test the day of surgery

It is important to note any bleeding problems or infections in the past as well any previous surgical or noninvasive procedures. Asking about previous scars can help ascertain how a patient heals and can elicit any previous surgical procedures.

Physical exam

The physical exam may be performed with the patient standing to assess for baseline irregularities and asymmetry. Asymmetries should be noted, highlighted, and explained to the patient, who may or may not be aware of such. The patient should be either completely undressed or given a disposable bikini undergarment, which has no elastic constriction. This avoids any distortion of the natural contour of the area and any artifactual step-offs when evaluating the patient. The pinch test, which is done by pinching the area of interest between the thumb and index finger, is often used both pre-surgically and during the operation. An area of adiposity where the surgeon can pinch at least an inch suggests an area where LAL can be effectively performed. A pinch of less than one inch may

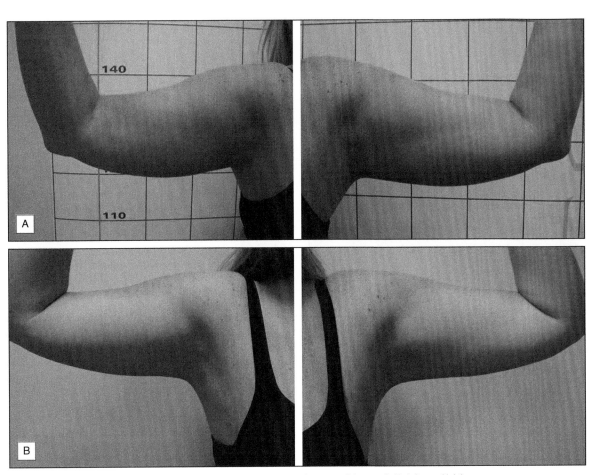

Figure 10.3 (A) Before and **(B)** 3 months after laser-assisted lipolysis to the arms; right arm (left), left arm (right)

indicate lack of sufficient fat to suction and increased risk of postoperative irregularities.

Baseline body weight as well as calculated BMI may be recorded. It is important to inform the patient that these parameters may not change post-procedure since liposuction is not a weight-reducing procedure. Circumferential measurements of the area being evaluated (bilateral thighs, hips, or waist) may be more likely to change post-procedure.

Skin laxity may also be assessed during the physical exam as this can be targeted and improved by LAL. Though it may tighten the dermal layer and therefore improve skin tone, LAL may not be able to create a completely flat, washboard appearance, which some patients may be expecting. To assess skin elasticity, the surgeon can perform the 'snap test' where the skin is gently pinched between the thumb and the index finger and then released. If there is an instantaneous recoil to rest position, this indicates good elasticity, and therefore a favorable potential response to LAL. If, however, there is slow recoil or no recoil at all, this indicates poor elasticity. Such patients may be made aware that they may be more likely to have residual skin folds after LAL. Other indications that

textural skin abnormalities or incomplete skin retraction may be post-procedure problems include the preoperative presence of cellulitic areas, dimples, larger depressions, excessive striae, and inelastic hanging skin folds.

Baseline photography

Appropriate imaging pre-treatment facilitates gauging improvement post-treatment as patients and physicians may not recall pre-surgical conditions many months later. Photography and imaging of adiposities can be easily altered by angle, lighting and shadowing, therefore these parameters are ideally standardized. Having a uniform background, fixing the patient position, and keeping constant the distance at which the image is taken can make for excellent quality images. Overhead or tangential illumination of the areas may be used to better visualize the surface area. Photographs may be taken with the patient standing and muscles relaxed. A total body photograph as well as multiple close-up photos of the individual areas can be obtained at the same time, with the former placing the latter in context. Subsequently, and before surgery, these images can be shown to the patient in order to

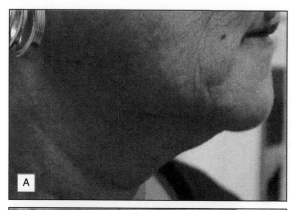

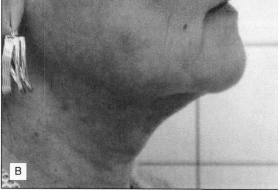

Figure 10.4 (A) Before and **(B)** 3 months after laser-assisted lipolysis to the submental and jowl area

initiate a frank discussion about the outcomes that are realistically possible.

Pearl 4

Use a standard black background for taking all photos. This will help to standardize images.

Use standard paper undergarments when taking photos to avoid distortion by waistbands and elastic banding.

Another option for imaging is a three-dimensional imaging system. While not necessary and inherently more costly, this technology can dramatically highlight post-procedure changes. The technology uses stereo-paired cameras to map out surface features. This technique is more resistant to inadvertent subject movement and also partially negates the effects of ambient room lightening. The imaging software additionally calculates the surface height and volume change within the treatment area.

Treatment course

LAL is performed in a manner similar to traditional or power-assisted liposuction and preparation can likewise be quite similar. Informed consent is obtained before com-

mencement. A urine pregnancy test may be performed on the day of surgery to confirm that the patient is not pregnant. Some physicians may prefer to dose oral antibiotics 24 hours before or at the time of tumescent infusion. The antibiotic is routinely one that covers the most common contaminating pathogen, *Staphylococcus aureus*. Some physicians offer the patient oral lorazepam 1–2 mg, or diazepam 5–10 mg at the time of surgery; in some instances, oral clonidine 0.1 mg on the day of the procedure may be administered if the patient's blood pressure is stable and above 100/70 mmHg in order to prevent epinephrine-induced tachycardia.

LAL is typically performed under local tumescent anesthesia alone, or supplemented with intravenous sedation, intramuscular pain medication, or epidural block. Some physicians perform a modified version of the procedure under general anesthesia.

Once marked, the patient is brought to the operating room or surgical suite and prepped widely, with the sterile area encompassing the surgical site area and proceeding well beyond to avoid inadvertent contamination. Usually either Betadine® (Becton Dickinson, Franklin Lakes, NJ) or Hibiclens® (Regent Medical, Norcross, GA) is the prep chemical. Skin cleansing is often done with the patient in the standing position. The patient may then be placed on the operating table upon the sterile draping. External pneumatic compression devices such as Venodyne® (Columbus, Mississippi) are occasionally also used on the legs, but this is not common or required.

Entry points are made in well-selected positions that provide overlapping access to the treatment site, and are also ergonomically positioned for optimal hand-positioning during treatment. The precise selection of sites is contingent on the area being treated. Multiple small entry points are typically favored over fewer larger diameter entry sites. This approach allows for suctioning of a given area from multiple points, thus allowing a smooth final contour, and smaller entry points also heal more quickly and less noticeably. A small #11 blade incision can be used to create entry points. Alternatively, a 1.5 mm or 2 mm punch biopsy tool may be employed, and it has been suggested that the resulting small wounds may heal particularly well (Fig. 10.1).

Pearl 5

Entry points for abdominal treatment can be hidden within the umbilicus.

All entry points should be discussed with the patient beforehand to ensure patient satisfaction.

Tumescent anesthesia

Subcutaneous infiltration of warmed Klein's tumescent solution is usually the preferred method of anesthesia for these authors. Typical Klein's solution contains 500–1000 mg lidocaine, 1 mg epinephrine and 12.5 mL of

8.4% sodium bicarbonate per 1 L of normal saline. This makes a buffered solution containing approximately 0.05% to 0.1%, respectively, of lidocaine and 1 : 1 000 000 units of epinephrine. In some cases, it may be preferable to use an intermediate concentration, a 0.075% lidocaine solution, which consists of 750 mg of lidocaine. Conservative dosing parameters are between 35 and 45 mg/kg of lidocaine though doses up to 55 mg/kg have been shown to be safe.[12] Warming the solution may help prevent drops in core body temperature after it is infused. The amount of anesthesia required depends on the size and anatomic location of the area being treated. The endpoint of anesthetic infusion is firm induration. Caution is advised to not over-infuse, which can lead to compression of vital structures in areas such as the neck. The tumescence is allowed to sit for at least 15 to 30 minutes, and as long as 1 hour, to allow for maximum diffusion into the intercellular space and vasoconstriction induction by epinephrine.

Pearl 6

The area around the umbilicus may require more anesthesia as it may not become as easily anesthetized as other areas.

Laser application and method

Prior to laser use, the patient and operators should all be wearing laser safety goggles with the appropriate optical density for the wavelength being used. Laser energy is conducted via an optical fiber usually measuring 600–1000 mm in diameter. This is housed within a cannula that is about 1–2 mm in diameter. Variations occur across different laser platforms created by different manufacturers so it is important to understand the specific operational properties of the device being used. All current systems are designed so that the laser fiber tip extends beyond the end of the cannula by 2–3 mm. This causes the laser to come into direct contact with adipose tissue, thereby permitting direct activity of the laser energy on the adipose tissue.

The optical fiber conducts both the therapeutic infrared wavelength and a helium–neon aiming beam at 634 nm. This beam is easily visualized and helps the physician precisely localize the fiber tip, including the depth of the laser fiber. If the beam becomes difficult to see, this could signify that the tip is in a relatively deeper tissue plane.

Since there are many different devices available, the physician should become familiar with each particular device he or she is likely to use in a clinical context (Table 10.2). The 1064 nm and 1320 nm wavelengths have different absorption characteristics. The 1320 nm wavelength has a higher coefficient of absorption in water than the 1064 nm wavelength, and so is associated with decreased scattering. Most of the energy delivered from a 1320 nm wavelength fiber will be absorbed in the area around the tip and it will also produce more dermal

Table 10.2 Devices used for laser application

Laser platform	Medium	Wavelength
SmoothLipo®: Eleme	Diode	920 nm
SlimLipo™: Palomar	Diode	924 nm; 975 nm
Lipotherme™: Osyris	Diode	980 nm
SmartLipo: Cynosure	Nd:YAG	1064 nm
LipoLite™: Syneron	Nd:YAG	1064 nm
ProLipo™: Sciton	Nd:YAG	1064 nm; 1319 nm
CoolLipo™: CoolTouch	Nd:YAG	1320 nm
SmartLipo MPX™: Cynosure	Nd:YAG	1064 nm; 1320 nm
SmartLipo Triplex: Cynosure	Nd:YAG	1064 nm; 1320 nm; 1440 nm

collagen remodeling. The 1064 nm has better absorption by hemoglobin and will permit more diffuse thermal spread and heating.

Some LAL devices combine multiple wavelengths while others combine multiple modalities. One device, CoolTouch® (Syneron, Roseville, CA), combines a laser fiber with an aspiration suction cannula. Other platforms have a motion-sensing feedback handpiece (Cynosure®), which will stop firing the device if the speed at which the laser fiber is moved drops below a predetermined threshold. The purpose is to prevent bulk heating by an accumulation of thermal energy, which can result in burns. The duration of laser activity needed for efficacy is dependent on certain variables including the area being treated, thickness of tissue, and volume of adipose targeted. The laser fiber is initially used to treat the deep subcutaneous fat layer in an effort to debulk this area. Once this is accomplished, the laser fiber can be directed into the superficial fat layer, closer to the dermis, to induce skin tightening. It is important during this latter part of the procedure that the fiber not be placed too superficially under the dermis for a prolonged period as this can cause thermal burns and cutaneous necrosis. Since adipose is known to be a good heat insulator, it is important to keep the laser fiber moving evenly and with consistent speed while firing. The cannula should be moved back and forth in a fanlike motion arcing about the entry point (see video). Care should be made not to keep re-entering the same tunnel made by the previous pass as this can cause excessive energy deposition. Also it is important not to entirely withdraw the laser fiber from the entry point while firing as this can cause thermal burns at the entry point. During treatment an infrared thermometer either external to the apparatus or housed within the laser device can be used to monitor tissue temperatures. Surface temperatures not exceeding 38 °C to 40 °C and internal temperatures around 47 °C (not exceeding 50 °C) are safe parameters to guide treatment. External cold packs can also be used to decrease surface temperatures and prevent excessive collateral thermal damage. The authors recommend using the pinch test to ensure that the areas being treated are uniformly thick. Treatment can be concluded when an inch can no longer be pinched, the entire treatment area is of equal thickness, and the desired contour has been achieved. An additional endpoint that can be used to guide treatment is the energy delivered. While there are no preset treatment parameters, Reynaud and colleagues published their recommended cumulative energies for different areas: knee, 8100 J; hip, 14 600 J; inner thigh, 10 400 J; chin, 11 700 J; arm, 12 800 J; buttock roll, 13 100 J; back, 21 900 J; abdomen, 24 600 J.[13] Some physicians also combine LAL with traditional aspiration or power-assisted liposuction. This can be done to remove the aspirate or to further contour and remove adiposities. If suctioning is performed, the operating physicians may wish to avoid being as aggressive as they might be if suctioning were performed without laser, as this precaution may help minimize the risk of contour irregularities.

To avoid complications and achieve successful results, various clinical endpoints should be considered in conjunction with physician judgment. Physicians should not persist in trying to deposit a certain preplanned amount of energy if tissue temperatures are becoming excessive. Also, to avoid excessive lipolysis, the tissue may be continually palpated with the nondominant hand until it becomes less dense and the desired thickness is reached.

Postoperative compression garments may be utilized, with the duration of application at the physician's discretion. We recommend using such compression for at least 7 days. The garments should not be overly constrictive such that numbness results. Garments appear to be useful to reduce swelling and improve skin redraping. We also recommend refraining from exercise for about 1 week.

Expected outcomes including supporting data from prior studies

Laser-assisted lipolysis has been studied and used with several different laser systems. In 2003, Badin and co-workers first reported successfully treating 245 patients with a 1064 nm Nd:YAG laser. The authors used a wet infiltration technique rather than tumescent anesthesia; however, they claimed that due to the small cannula size and unique laser–tissue effects, laser lipolysis was less traumatic than conventional liposuction and led to improved skin retraction.[9]

Badin then compared laser-assisted liposuction with liposuction without laser assistance. Two areas of the left flank in the patient were treated with 1000 J and 3000 J, and compared with the right flank, which was treated with conventional tumescent liposuction. Histologic evaluation of the laser-treated tissue revealed areas of tumefaction and lysis, features which were not observed with tumescent liposuction alone. Additionally, the laser treated side had less intense bleeding. The degree of tumefaction and lysis was proportional to the total energy accumulated.[5]

The authors postulated that the laser's ability to cause microangiopathic coagulation might reduce bleeding and allow for the safe removal of larger volumes of fat relative to conventional liposuction.

Goldman reported his results after treating the submental area of 82 patients using laser liposuction with a 1064 nm Nd:YAG laser. Biopsies were obtained immediately following treatment as well as 40 days post-treatment. Histologic evaluation of the biopsies obtained 40 days later revealed evidence of new collagen formation and decreased adipocytes. As there was no control arm to the study, it remains to be determined whether these changes (i.e. the new collagen formation) were related to the effects of laser or a healing response to liposuction itself.[2]

A study by Kim and Geronemus used magnetic resonance imaging (MRI) to quantify the volume of fat reduction from laser lipolysis.[14] The authors treated 30 patients with the 1064 nm Nd:YAG laser without aspiration in the submental area, upper arm, and thigh and obtained pre-procedural and 3-months' post-procedure MRI scans of 10 subjects. They noted a statistically significant average fat reduction of 16.7% and showed that a dose–response relationship existed between energy applied and degree of lipolysis. This dose–response relationship was subsequently characterized by a mathematical optical-thermal-damage model that showed a 10 cm^3 volume reduction after 6600 J of energy, with a linear relationship between energy applied and fat volume reduction, irrespective of wavelength used. Furthermore, the authors determined that subcutaneous temperatures of 48–50 °C are sufficient to induce skin tightening.[15]

Rho and colleagues evaluated the efficacy of the 1064 nm Nd:YAG laser in the treatment of gynecomastia and pseudogynecomastia. Five male subjects were enrolled in a controlled split-breast trial. One breast was treated with laser lipolysis (without aspiration), with the control arm of the study being the untreated contralateral breast. Results were evaluated using computed tomography and ultrasound imaging as well as chest circumference. The investigators found decreased chest circumference and decreased thickness of the treated breast 8 weeks postoperatively, with high patient satisfaction and minimal side effects (ecchymosis, pain, edema).[16]

Dudelzak et al.[17] evaluated the effectiveness of laser lipolysis for fat reduction in the arms. The authors treated 20 female subjects with a 1064 nm Nd:YAG laser. Cumulative energy per treated arm ranged from 7112 to 12 026 J, and the liquefied fat was removed through a liposuction cannula in half of the subjects. Eighty percent of patients experienced a decrease in upper arm circumference. Results were similar regardless of whether aspiration was performed.[17]

Sun and colleagues treated 35 Asian patients with localized adiposis using a 1064 nm Nd:YAG laser with a 1 mm cannula, with and without aspiration.[18] Twenty-eight of 35 patients were satisfied with the improvement of their adiposity. The authors noted that the more fibrous and compact the tissues contained in the adiposis, the higher the laser energy density needed for treatment per unit volume, with the nuchal region requiring the most followed by the face, mental region, upper arm, and abdomen, respectively. However, due to prolongation of the operative time required for laser lipolysis, the authors suggest that laser lipolysis may be better indicated for treatment of smaller areas of adiposis rather than larger areas like the abdomen.

Subsequent to multiple studies which demonstrated safety and efficacy using a 1064 nm Nd:YAG laser, Reynaud and colleagues investigated the efficacy of laser lipolysis using the 980 nm diode laser with and without subsequent aspiration in a study of 334 subjects.[13] Mean cumulative energy required was found to be area-dependent, ranging from 2200 J (knee) to 51 000 J (abdomen).[13] Contour correction and skin retraction were observed almost immediately in most patients. Furthermore, there was high patient satisfaction with the procedure (58% were 'very satisfied' and another 22% were 'satisfied') and a good safety profile was maintained.[13]

Another laser in the armamentarium of laser-assisted lipolysis devices is a dual-wavelength diode laser (Slim-Lipo™, Palomar Medical Technologies Inc., Burlington, MA) that operates at 924 nm and 975 nm wavelengths, with subsequent aspiration. The safety and efficacy of this laser was investigated by Weiss and Beasley who treated 19 subjects. Outcomes were measured according to investigator and subject self-assessments. Good to excellent improvement was reported in all treated subjects and no significant adverse events were seen.[19]

More recently, laser-assisted lipolysis has included combination or sequential laser treatment during the procedure (e.g. SmartLipo MPX™ (Cynosure, Westford, MA), a sequentially firing 1064 nm/1320 nm Nd:YAG laser). McBean and Katz evaluated skin tightening and histologic changes in 20 patients treated using a sequentially firing 1064 nm/1320 nm Nd:YAG laser with and without aspiration. Independent observers found 76–100% improvement in 85% of subjects on photographic documentation. India ink tattoo maps demonstrated an 18% decrease in surface area at the treated sites. Histologically, the authors observed parallel bundles of collagen consistent with neocollagenesis.[20] No adverse events were reported. Sasaki and Tevez also reported on their experience in treating 75 patients with the dual 1064 nm/1320 nm Nd:YAG laser and found an 80%, patient-reported, degree of improvement at 2–3 months.[21]

Woodhall and colleagues conducted comparison studies of the safety and efficacy of 1064 nm, 1320 nm, and dual 1064 nm/1320 nm Nd:YAG laser-assisted lipolysis. In their first investigation, one arm was randomized to treatment with a subcutaneous 1064 nm Nd:YAG laser and showed no significant improvement over tumescent liposuction alone. In the second study, half of the treatment area was randomized to receive the 1064 nm versus the 1320 nm system, followed by aspiration. The authors were unable to show significant improvement with either

system. The third study treated patients using a combined 1064 nm/1320 nm multiplex laser system at multiple sites and showed resulting improvement in skin laxity and fat reduction.[22]

Alexiades-Armenakas also performed a three-arm study evaluating laser-assisted lipolysis and minimally invasive skin tightening using the 1064 nm and 1319 nm Nd:YAG lasers, independently and in combination.[23] Twelve subjects with excessive submental fat and neck laxity were treated. Effectiveness of fat removal was similar for the three wavelength combinations, and excellent laxity reduction was reported for all three study arms, with no statistically significant differences between them. During the study, direct in situ temperature feedback was used to maintain a uniform target temperature of 45–48 °C in the targeted plane and avoid thermal burns, which did not occur.[23]

Laser-assisted lipolysis has also been applied safely and successfully to the treatment of unwanted fat of less traditional anatomic areas including knees,[24] ankles,[25] breasts for the treatment of gynecomastia,[26] and the cervicodorsal area for treatment of the underlying fat pad (buffalo hump in a patient with HIV lipodystrophy).[27]

Very few comparative randomized controlled trials have evaluated the increased efficacy of laser-assisted liposuction over traditional tumescent liposuction. Prado et al.[28] conducted a split-body randomized double-blind trial of 25 patients comparing 1064 nm Nd:YAG and suction-assisted liposuction. The authors were unable to demonstrate an improved cosmetic outcome on the laser-assisted side, irrespective of the treatment site.[28] Sasaki conducted a small study to quantify tissue tightening and contraction after 1064 nm/1320 nm LAL compared to traditional liposuction alone. Using three-dimensional imaging (Vectra, Canfield Scientific, NJ) skin contraction was measured at 3 months. A slight increase in skin contraction (3.6% above baseline) was noted in areas treated with liposuction or deep lasing plus liposuction. Slightly more skin contraction (4.2% from baseline) was seen after the combination of shallow lasing, traditional liposuction, and deep lasing.[29]

Safety

Laser-assisted lipolysis has been studied extensively with respect to adverse events and complications, using the various laser devices on the market. A retrospective analysis of 537 procedures by Katz and McBean revealed a low complication rate.[30] There were five local complications (one skin infection and four skin burns), and no systemic complications. The local complication rate was less than 1%, and touch-ups were required only 19 times (3.5%).[30] All of the burns were successfully treated with topical emollients or antibacterial ointments and the infection resolved without sequelae.

The overall safety profile of laser-assisted liposuction is similar to that of traditional tumescent liposuction, with the additional risk of skin burns, which may be associated with a lack of direct in situ temperature feedback during the procedure. Skin burns have been reported in large clinical studies as well as single case reports, including a case report of a patient who underwent laser lipolysis blepharoplasty using the EyeTight® (LaserTight, Cherry Hill, NJ) 980 nm diode laser and developed a full-thickness dermal burn.[31] DiBernardo and colleagues found a correlation between greater temperature and tissue injury. A surface temperature as low as 47 °C was associated with epidermal and dermal injury and therefore it was recommended that the surface temperature is maintained below 42 °C in order to avoid burns and scarring.[32]

Chia and Theodorou evaluated 1000 cases of laser-assisted lipolysis using the 1064 nm and/or 1320 nm Nd:YAG lasers and reported the following complications: two patients treated for neck adiposities sustained partial-thickness burns, one patient had a burn requiring treatment with steroid injections and scar revision, one patient had a postoperative hematoma, and two infections were treated successfully with a course of antibiotics. A total of 73 patients (7.3%) underwent secondary or touch-up procedures for further fat resection.[33]

Licata et al. reported on their experience using a 1540 nm diode laser for suction-assisted laser lipolysis on 230 patients. Among the observations were 43 cases of postoperative edema and 20 cases of ecchymoses, all of which resolved within 1 week.[34] Collawn reported on her experience using the Smartlipo MPX™ (1064 nm and 1320 nm) (Cynosure, Westford, MA, USA) for body and face contouring on 72 patients. No complications were seen on the face and only one blister developed on the thigh, which healed with a topical antibiotic.[35]

Other less commonly reported adverse events have also been described. Sasaki and Tevez reported that approximately 5% of patients developed nodularity within 6 weeks of treatment.[21] Nodules were successfully managed using external ultrasound treatments. Other reported adverse events included temporary ecchymoses and transient localized sponginess in the abdomens of three patients, which resolved spontaneously within 1 month.[21]

Case reports of laser-assisted liposuction resulting in adverse events such as skin burns, contour irregularity and cobblestoning have been described.[36,37] The loose excess skin of the neck is particularly prone to developing a cobblestoned appearance if inappropriately treated with excessive energies.

The systemic implications of lipolysis have been addressed by monitoring postoperative lipid levels. Mordon and colleagues investigated serum lipid changes following laser lipolysis using the 980 nm diode laser (Osyris Medical, Hellemmes, France).[8] No change in serum cholesterol or triglyceride levels was detected following treatment at various energy levels at 1 month follow-up.

Some techniques geared at preventing rapid accumulation of thermal energy localized to one area can be employed to prevent skin burns. Methods include moving the laser handpiece at a rate of at least 1 cm/s, keeping the tip in the correct tissue plane (i.e. placing the fiber-optic cannula in the deep and intermediate subcutaneous spaces), and exercising extreme caution at certain anatomic sites. Areas that may be at greater risk for thermal injury include points of natural curvature or bony prominences. In such areas, the laser may need to be intermittently switched off as needed to minimize the risk of a burn. Another way to potentially prevent inadvertent burns is to monitor the temperature of the skin with a thermal scanning device that measures cutaneous temperature. Some devices are equipped with a thermal probe at the laser fiber tip with which to monitor internal temperature. In some cases these cause the device to cease firing if temperature levels reach a preset threshold.

Although numerous studies have shown the overall safety of LAL, a good understanding of laser–tissue interactions and skin and subcutaneous tissue anatomy increases the likelihood of safe and effective use in a given patient. A thorough preoperative patient evaluation can help determine if laser-assisted lipolysis is the treatment of choice for a particular patient's needs and expectations. If performed inappropriately or sometimes by chance alone at certain anatomic areas, laser-assisted lipolysis can result in poor outcomes, including epidermal and dermal thermal injury, blistering, burns, cobblestoning, seroma and hematoma formation, and infection.

Multi-modality procedures

Since the efficacy and safety of laser lipolysis were demonstrated in initial studies, the popularity of laser lipolysis has grown, as have the indications and uses, including combination treatment with other modalities. Goldman and colleagues combined laser lipolysis with autologous fat transplantation to treat 52 female patients with Curri grade III–IV cellulite.[38] The authors used a 1064 nm Nd:YAG laser under tumescent anesthesia, applying laser energy in both the superficial subdermal plane (to induce neocollagenesis), then the deeper subcutaneous plane (to cause adipose reduction). Depressed areas of cellulite received autologous fat injections with overcorrection of approximately 10% to 15%. Patient 1-year postoperative self-assessment scores showed a good outcome in 54% of cases and an excellent outcome in 31%.[38] However, the study lacked a control arm to compare the combination technique to autologous fat transplantation alone or tumescent liposuction without autologous fat transplantation.

Aboelatta et al.[39] investigated combining laser-assisted liposuction using a 1320 nm Nd:YAG laser with a short pulse duration of 100 µs (CoolLipo™, New Star Lasers, CoolTouch Inc., Roseville, CA, USA) followed immediately by abdominoplasty. Skin temperature was controlled not to exceed 34 °C. Although the authors found that patients who underwent laser liposuction with abdominoplasty had statistically significant improvement in skin tightness and skin contour compared to those receiving conventional liposuction with abdominoplasty, this group also had an increased frequency of adverse events. Three out of 12 patients developed a seroma and three out of 12 developed skin necrosis or dehiscence.[39]

Collawn described using a multi-laser approach to achieve reduction of adiposity, skin tightening, and reduction of rhytides. She reported her experience combining laser-assisted liposuction (Smartlipo (1064 nm or MPX with combined 1064 nm and 1320 nm)) and nonablative (1440 nm, 1320 nm) fractional CO_2 laser treatment.[40]

Conclusion

LAL has become an integral tool in body contouring and for the treatment of localized adiposity. LAL either alone or in combination with aspiration liposuction can produce significant and lasting adipose reduction as well as skin tightening. Added benefits of LAL compared with liposuction alone may include decreased bruising, decreased blood loss, faster recovery time, and increased skin tightening and contraction. Proper pre-surgical patient evaluation and selection along with a thorough discussion of realistic expectations can make for a successful treatment course. With new devices coming to market at a rapid pace, it is important for the operating physician to understand the fundamentals of LAL as well as the specific parameters of each device. Devices with combined wavelengths or modalities may augment clinical practice but may also increase the risk for potential complications. It is prudent to exercise proper clinical judgment when utilizing any of these modalities.

CASE STUDY 1 (See Fig. 10.2)

A 38-year-old female presented with abdominal adiposities that had not improved with regular dieting. She reported maintaining a consistent weight over the past 5 years, and exercising about once a week. She had a caesarian section with the birth of her child, but reports no history of abdominal hernias, no keloids or hypertrophic scarring, and no other medical problems or drug allergies. She has not previously had any invasive or noninvasive adipose treatments. On physical exam, there are localized adiposities in the upper and lower abdominal area. While striae are seen on the bilateral flanks/hip roll, there is no excessive skin laxity, with a negative snap test in which the skin quickly regains its original form. Preoperative blood tests were ordered, including complete metabolic profile with liver profile, complete blood count with differential, prothrombin time, partial thromboplastin time, HIV antibody, hepatitis C antibody, and beta-human chorionic gonadotrophin. All values were within normal limits. The patient was given a prescription for cephalexin 500 mg orally twice a day starting 1 day before surgery and continuing for 7 days post-operation. An abdominal compression garment was ordered for her as well.

Treatment

On the day of surgery, standardized photos were obtained and circumferential measurements were recorded. The patient's blood pressure and pulse were also recorded. A urine pregnancy test was performed to reconfirm that the patient was not currently pregnant. After local injection of 1%

lidocaine with epinephrine, entry points were made in the upper and lower umbilicus with a 1.5 mm punch biopsy tool to access the upper and lower abdomen, respectively. Two more entry points were created in the bilateral lower abdomen at the waistline. A total of 1 L of tumescent anesthesia comprising 0.075% Klein's formula was infiltrated and allowed to sit for 30 minutes.

When treatment commenced, a 1320 nm laser fiber at power 10–15 W was first used in the deeper adipose layer to debulk adiposities. Treatment was guided by pinching the adiposities between the thumb and index finger and feeling decreased bulk as the procedure continued. After this, the laser fiber was positioned in the subcutaneous fat layer just below the dermal junction to initiate the skin tightening portion of the procedure. This again was guided by maintaining a level plane and an even area of pinched fat. After the laser lipolysis was completed, power-assisted liposuction was performed to remove the lased aspirate as well as to remove additional fat for fine contouring of the upper and lower abdomen. Approximately 800 mL of aspirate was extracted, with about 500 mL of that being fat and the remainder serosanguinous supernatant. An abdominal compression garment was given for the patient to wear continuously for 1 week and then during the day only for 3 weeks more. Postoperative photos were obtained at 3 months (Fig. 10.2).

CASE STUDY 2 (See Fig. 10.3)

A 45-year-old female was seen for evaluation and treatment of upper arm adiposities and skin laxity. The patient stated that she was not happy with the appearance of the upper arms despite a regular exercise program. Prior medical history and results of routine blood tests did not reveal any problems. On pinch test, the patient was noted to have mild skin laxity, and the risks of residual laxity after treatment were discussed with her.

Treatment

On the day of surgery, after routine measurements and tests, entry points were made in the upper arm, just distal to the axillary vault, and also just proximal to the elbow, both with a 1.5 mm punch biopsy tool. These sites were selected to allow bidirectional access to the upper arm. Tumescent anesthesia comprising 250 mL of 0.075% Klein's formula was infiltrated.

Treatment was then started with use of a 1320 nm laser fiber, set at a power of 10 W, in the deeper adipose layer to debulk adiposities. While making tunnels with the laser device, and maintaining a continuous fan-like movement, particular caution was exercised in the area of the axillary vault. Here, it was important to not tunnel too deeply as the brachial nerve plexus courses under the axilla.

After this, the laser fiber was repositioned for skin tightening purposes, and this was then followed by power liposuction for further debulking and contouring. Approximately 250 mL of aspirate was removed from each arm with about 150 mL of that being adipose tissue. Postoperative instructions and course were routine (Fig. 10.3).

References

1. ASAPS. Cosmetic Surgery National Data Bank Statistics, 2010.
2. Goldman A. Submental Nd:YAG laser-assisted liposuction. Lasers Surg Med 2006;38(3):181–4.
3. Anderson RR, Farinelli W, Laubach H, et al. Selective photothermolysis of lipid-rich tissues: a free electron laser study. Lasers Surg Med 2006;38(10):913–19.
4. Apfelberg D. Laser-assisted liposuction may benefit surgeons, patients. Clin Laser Mon 1992;10(12):193–4.
5. Badin AZ, Gondek LB, Garcia MJ, et al. Analysis of laser lipolysis effects on human tissue samples obtained from liposuction. Aesthetic Plast Surg 2005;29(4):281–6.
6. Ichikawa K, Miyasaka M, Tanaka R, et al. Histologic evaluation of the pulsed Nd:YAG laser for laser lipolysis. Lasers Surg Med 2005;36(1):43–6.
7. Mordon S, Eymard-Maurin AF, Wassmer B, et al. Histologic evaluation of laser lipolysis: pulsed 1064-nm Nd:YAG laser versus CW 980-nm diode laser. Aesthet Surg J 2007;27(3): 263–8.
8. Mordon S, Wassmer B, Rochon P, et al. Serum lipid changes following laser lipolysis. J Cosmet Laser Ther 2009;11(2): 74–7.
9. Badin AZ, Moraes LM, Gondek L, et al. Laser lipolysis: flaccidity under control. Aesthetic Plast Surg 2002;26(5): 335–9.
10. DiBernardo BE, Reyes J. Evaluation of skin tightening after laser-assisted liposuction. Aesthet Surg J 2009;29(5):400–7.
11. Stebbins WG, Hanke CW, Petersen J. Novel method of minimally invasive removal of large lipoma after laser lipolysis with 980 nm diode laser. Dermatol Ther 2011;24(1):125–30.
12. Ostad A, Kageyama N, Moy RL. Tumescent anesthesia with a lidocaine dose of 55 mg/kg is safe for liposuction. Dermatol Surg 1996;22(11):921–7.
13. Reynaud JP, Skibinski M, Wassmer B, et al. Lipolysis using a 980-nm diode laser: a retrospective analysis of 534 procedures. Aesthetic Plast Surg 2009;33(1):28–36.
14. Kim KH, Geronemus RG. Laser lipolysis using a novel 1,064 nm Nd:YAG Laser. Dermatol Surg 2006;32(2):241–8, discussion 247.
15. Mordon SR, Wassmer B, Reynaud JP, et al. Mathematical modeling of laser lipolysis. Biomed Eng Online 2008;7:10.
16. Rho YK, Kim BJ, Kim MN, et al. Laser lipolysis with pulsed 1064 nm Nd:YAG laser for the treatment of gynecomastia. Int J Dermatol 2009;48(12):1353–9.
17. Dudelzak J, Hussain M, Goldberg DJ. Laser lipolysis of the arm, with and without suction aspiration: clinical and histologic changes. J Cosmet Laser Ther 2009;11(2):70–3.
18. Sun Y, Wu SF, Yan S, et al. Laser lipolysis used to treat localized adiposis: a preliminary report on experience with Asian patients. Aesthetic Plast Surg 2009;33(5):701–5.
19. Weiss RA, Beasley K. Laser-assisted liposuction using a novel blend of lipid- and water-selective wavelengths. Lasers Surg Med 2009;41(10):760–766.
20. McBean JC, Katz BE. A pilot study of the efficacy of a 1,064 and 1,320 nm sequentially firing Nd:YAG laser device for lipolysis and skin tightening. Lasers Surg Med 2009;41(10): 779–84.
21. Sasaki GH, Tevez A. Laser-assisted liposuction for facial and body contouring and tissue tightening: a 2-year experience with 75 consecutive patients. Semin Cutan Med Surg 2009;28(4): 226–35.
22. Woodhall KE, Saluja R, Khoury J, et al. A comparison of three separate clinical studies evaluating the safety and efficacy of laser-assisted lipolysis using 1,064, 1,320 nm, and a combined 1,064/1,320 nm multiplex device. Lasers Surg Med 2009; 41(10):774–8.
23. Alexiades-Armenakas M. Combination laser-assisted liposuction and minimally invasive skin tightening with temperature feedback for treatment of the submentum and neck. Dermatol Surg 2012;38(6):871–81.
24. Moreno-Moraga J, Trelles MA, Mordon S, et al. Laser-assisted lipolysis for knee remodelling: a prospective study in 30 patients. J Cosmet Laser Ther 2012;14(2):59–66.
25. Leclere FM, Moreno-Moraga J, Mordon S, et al. Laser-assisted lipolysis for cankle remodelling: a prospective study in 30 patients. Lasers Med Sci 2014;29(1):31–6.
26. Trelles MA, Mordon SR, Bonanad E, et al. Laser-assisted lipolysis in the treatment of gynecomastia: a prospective study in 28 patients. Lasers Med Sci 2013;28(2):375–82.
27. Onesti MG, Fioramonti P, Carella S, et al. Nd:YAG laser-assisted liposuction for an HIV patient. Aesthetic Plast Surg 2010;34(4):528–30.
28. Prado A, Andrades P, Danilla S, et al. A prospective, randomized, double-blind, controlled clinical trial comparing laser-assisted lipoplasty with suction-assisted lipoplasty. Plast Reconstr Surg 2006;118(4):1032–45.
29. Sasaki GH. Quantification of human abdominal tissue tightening and contraction after component treatments with 1064-nm/1320-nm laser-assisted lipolysis: clinical implications. Aesthet Surg J 2010;30(2):239–45.
30. Katz B, McBean J. Laser-assisted lipolysis: a report on complications. J Cosmet Laser Ther 2008;10(4):231–3.
31. Yu D, Biesman B, Khan JA. Bilateral eyelid dermal burn from subcutaneous diode laser lipolysis blepharoplasty. Lasers Surg Med 2009;41(9):609–11.
32. DiBernardo BE, Reyes J, Chen B. Evaluation of tissue thermal effects from 1064/1320-nm laser-assisted lipolysis and its clinical implications. J Cosmet Laser Ther 2009;11(2):62–9.
33. Chia CT, Theodorou SJ. 1,000 consecutive cases of laser-assisted liposuction and suction-assisted lipectomy managed with local anesthesia. Aesthetic Plast Surg 2012;36(4): 795–802.
34. Licata G, Agostini T, Fanelli G, et al. Lipolysis using a new 1540-nm diode laser: a retrospective analysis of 230 consecutive procedures. J Cosmet Laser Ther 2013;15(4): 184–92.
35. Collawn SS. Smartlipo MPX sculpting of the body and face. J Cosmet Laser Ther 2011;13(4):172–5.
36. Sasser C, Blum C, Kaplan J. Discussion of preoperative indications and postoperative complications following laser-assisted lipolysis by non-plastic surgeons. Plast Reconstr Surg 2012;130(3):497e–8e.
37. Blum CA, Sasser CG, Kaplan JL. Complications from laser-assisted liposuction performed by noncore practitioners. Aesthetic Plast Surg 2013;37(5):869–75.
38. Goldman A, Gotkin RH, Sarnoff DS, et al. Cellulite: a new treatment approach combining subdermal Nd:YAG laser lipolysis and autologous fat transplantation. Aesthet Surg J 2008;28(6):656–62.
39. Aboelatta YA, Abdelaal MM, Bersy NA. The effectiveness and safety of combining laser-assisted liposuction and abdominoplasty. Aesthetic Plast Surg 2013.
40. Collawn S. Skin tightening with fractional lasers, radiofrequency, Smartlipo. Ann Plast Surg 2010;64(5):526–9.

Injectable Fat-reducing Therapies: Fat Reduction

11

Nazanin Saedi, Adam M. Rotunda, Jeffrey S. Dover

Key Messages

- Adipocytolysis refers to the subcutaneous injection of chemicals, such as the detergent sodium deoxycholate, which ablates or lyses rather than shrinks fat cells

- Injection lipolysis, otherwise known as pharmaceutical lipoplasty, refers to the subcutaneous injection of compounds, such as the beta agonist, salmeterol xinafoate, which mobilizes triglyceride and reduces fat cell size without lysing or ablating the fat cell

- While there are currently no FDA-cleared injectable agents for fat reduction, two therapies with differing mechanisms of action, salmeterol xinafoate and sodium deoxycholate, have demonstrated promising outcomes in clinical trials

Introduction

Body contouring refers to optimizing the definition, smoothness, and shape of the human physique.[1] With the substantial rising demand for body contouring over the past decade, noninvasive methods for fat reduction have become increasingly available. Historically, the approach to body contouring has largely involved invasive procedures such as liposuction and abdominoplasty. Liposuction is one of the most popular cosmetic surgical procedure in the United States, but it is invasive (surgical) with attendant downtime and rare but potential risks, including complications from anesthesia, infection, embolism, and even death.

In recent years, increasing numbers of nonobese patients have been looking for body contouring procedures with minimal downtime and with minimal risk, even if they are not as effective as liposuction and may require multiple treatments. Currently available nonsurgical body contouring devices include cryolipolysis,[2] low level laser therapy,[3] low energy nonthermal ultrasound,[4] and high intensity focused ultrasound.[5] While these devices have demonstrated safety, their efficacy across a wide range of patients is variable. Furthermore, the level of scientific rigor needed for FDA clearance of devices – small, open

label, primarily safety-oriented clinical studies – does not approach the level of rigor required for a medication; that is, large, randomized, double blind, placebo-controlled studies with stringent safety and efficacy endpoints. Conducting pharmaceutical drug registration studies takes a decade or more and costs well up to $100 000 000. While this has thus far limited the number of injectable, minimally invasive therapies in the therapeutic pipeline, it ensures that those therapies that make it to market are safe and efficacious.

As of this writing (2014), two subcutaneously injected medications, salmeterol xinafoate (SX) and sodium deoxycholate, are under investigation in FDA-regulated clinical trials and show great promise.

Pearl 1

Injection lipolysis (or pharmaceutical lipoplasty) refers to the subcutaneous injections of compounds that mobilize triglyceride and reduce fat cell size without lysing or ablating the fat cell, such as the beta agonist salmeterol xinafoate.

Background and mechanism of action

Fat cell ablation

Injectable fat-reducing techniques were first described by Brazilian dermatologist Patricia Rittes MD, when she reported reduction of infraorbital fat using direct, transcutaneous injection with Lipostabil® (Sanofi-Aventis, Paris, France).[6] Lipostabil is a solution consisting of soy-derived phosphatidylcholine (5%) with its solvent sodium deoxycholate (2.5%) in sterile water. In this initial report, 30 patients were injected with a total of 0.4 mL Lipostabil (50 mg/mL phosphatidylcholine (PC), 25 mg/mL deoxycholate (DC)) under each eye, and the treatments were 15 days apart. Most patients (22/30) in the study only had one or two treatments. Based on subjective data, all patients experienced reduction of infraorbital fat herniation, and the results persisted after observing them for 2 years. Rittes' report inspired numerous clinicians to request and use compounded PC (which indeed also contained DC) as a minimally invasive fat loss procedure for trunk and extremity fat. This practice lead to relatively widespread use of treatments using pharmacy compounded PC/DC, called Lipodissolve, which was unregulated and as a result was wrought with controversy. Tighter regulation and additional scientific investigation aimed at purifying and simplifying the injectable formulation led to a diminution of PC-containing compounded medications and focus on its solvent, DC.

Originally, it was thought that PC was the active fat-reducing ingredient in Lipostabil. Furthermore, PC was hypothesized to induce a cascade of intracellular signals that lead to apoptosis, or it directly lyses fat cell membranes, emulsifies triglycerides, upregulates lipoprotein lipase, and facilitates transit of triglycerides across cell membranes.[7,8] None of these theories could be proven experimentally or clinically. However, the discovery that DC, the solvent of PC, rather than PC itself, was the agent responsible for fat reduction changed the landscape of clinical investigation.[9] Ironically, PC was found to be a bystander rather than an active ingredient in the original Lipostabil studies and Lipodissolve treatments.

Numerous studies have supported the original observation that DC was the primary agent responsible for fat cell destruction. Gupta et al.[10] demonstrated that DC alone and PC/DC are cytotoxic to cultured adipocytes, endothelial cells, fibroblasts, and skeletal muscle cells. DC alone produced cell death and cell lysis in vitro (keratinocytes) and ex vivo (pig adipose tissue) equal to that produced by the PC/DC combination. These results were confirmed by the work of Rotunda et al.[9] that PC was the fat-reducing agent since it was again demonstrated that DC produced nonspecific cell lysis independent of PC. Klein et al.[11] further demonstrated that decrease in fat volume after Lipostabil injections is likely attributable to the detergent effect of DC.

Physiologically, deoxycholic acid is a secondary bile acid produced by intestinal bacteria after the release of primary bile acids in the liver. Chemically, DC is a detergent (Fig. 11.1). Detergents or surfactants are amphipathic molecules that contain both polar and nonpolar groups that are soluble in water. DC disrupts the integrity of biological membranes by introducing their polar hydroxyl groups into the cell membrane's phospholipid bilayer hydrophobic core. Once in contact with cell membranes, its amphipathic tendencies cause it to integrate into cell membranes. The process involves an 'attack' of the detergent on the membrane, solubilization of membrane-associated proteins, saturation of the membrane with detergent, and then finally, with increasing detergent concentration, membrane integrity breakdown, and solubilysis.[12–14] With high enough concentration, detergents fully saturate then destabilize cell membranes, which leads to solubilization and cell destruction (Fig. 11.2). Any detergent-based formulation elicits adipocyte lysis, and so it will not effectively stimulate adipocyte lipolysis, which is a process that requires a fully functioning, or viable, fat cell. In order to more accurately describe injectable methods that employ detergents to diminish fat, the term 'adipocytolysis' can be used.[15]

Pearl 2

Adipocytolysis refers to the subcutaneous injection of chemicals that ablate or lyse rather than shrink fat cells, such as the detergent sodium deoxycholate.

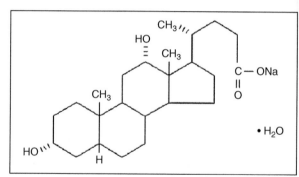

Figure 11.1 Chemical structure of sodium deoxycholate

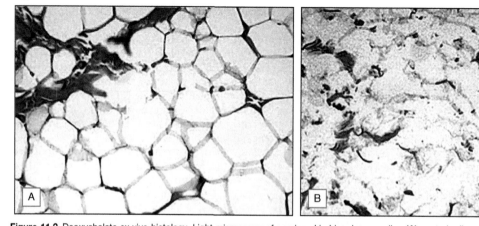

Figure 11.2 Deoxycholate ex vivo histology. Light microscopy of porcine skin biopsies revealing **(A)** control adipocytes and **(B)** adipocytes after deoxycholate injection (hematoxylin and eosin, original magnification ×20) *(from Rotunda AM, et al. Dermatol Surg 2004; 30:1001–8, with permission)*

Subcutaneously injected DC leads to tissue necrosis as a result of its cytotoxic, detergent effects on the cellular membranes. In vivo and ex vivo animal or human tissue exposed to DC demonstrate fat cell lysis, fat, muscle, and collagen necrosis; erythrocyte extravasation; a mixed infiltrate consisting of polymorphonuclear leukocytes, lymphocytes, macrophages; multinucleated giant cells, and fibrosis.[9,16,17]

As noted, in vitro, DC destroys nonadipose cells.[9,10] Since it has the capacity to destroy nonadipose cells, we need to explain how it can be selective for adipose tissue (Fig. 11.3). The ability of DC to lyse cells is inversely related to the amount of protein surrounding it and within tissue with which it comes into contact.[18] The presence of albumin appears to inhibit the cell lysing activity of DC. Albumin is found in high concentrations in vital tissue but low concentrations in fat, which can explain why injections of low dose DC into fat are relatively safe clinically.[19] This 'safety valve' effect of albumin on DC has fortunately made it an ideal candidate for subcutaneous fat injection.

At the time of this publication, there is a synthetic, purified (nonanimal derived) sodium deoxycholate, referred to experimentally as ATX-101 (KYTHERA Biopharmaceuticals, Calabasas, CA). ATX-101 is a low-dose formulation of a purified synthetic version of deoxycholic acid that causes focal adipocytolysis, which describes the destruction of adipocytes while leaving surrounding tissue largely unaffected. The resulting expected local tissue response involves macrophages eliminating cell debris and lipids from the treatment area, and the recruitment of fibroblasts, which are believed to be responsible for neocollagenesis. ATX-101 has completed Phase III clinical trials in the US and the European Union. The first indication of the treatment is for the reduction of submental fat (Fig. 11.4). Since there is no current FDA-approved injectable drug to reduce submental fat, this treatment may become a viable option for a growing, unmet need.

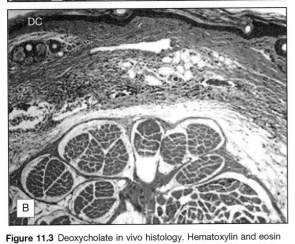

Figure 11.3 Deoxycholate in vivo histology. Hematoxylin and eosin staining of a mouse tail 20 days post-injection of **(A)** saline vehicle and **(B)** 0.5% deoxycholate showing necrosis and inflammatory infiltrate of the subcutaneous fat in the treated tail. The tissue architecture of the muscle and skin layers remains preserved in the treated tail, with no signs of necrosis and scant inflammation *(from Thuangtong R, et al. Dermatol Surg 2010; 36:899–908, with permission)*

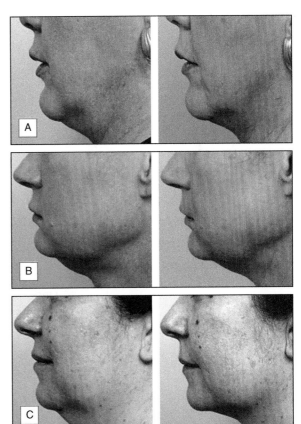

Figure 11.4 Profiles of patients treated before (left) and after (right) five monthly treatments with sodium dexycholate to the submental neck *(from Rotunda AM, et al. Dermatol Surg 2009; 35:792–803, with permission)*

Fat cell lipolysis

Whereas detergents work by causing focal adipocytolysis, other compounds, such as salmeterol xinafoate (SX), work by mobilizing intracellular triglyceride and reducing fat without lysing or ablating fat cells. The terms 'injection lipolysis' or 'pharmaceutical lipoplasty' refer to subcutaneous injections of compounds that mobilize and reduce fat without lysing or ablating cells.[20] The term lipolysis is used to describe hydrolysis or breakdown of lipids into constituent fatty acid and glycerol building blocks. Lipolysis can occur within adipocytes or within the vascular space of muscle and fat tissue, and is governed by hormone sensitive lipase and lipoprotein lipase. Medications (e.g. salmeterol, isoproterenol, etc.) and neurotransmitters (e.g. epinephrine, norepinephrine) that bind to specific adrenergic receptors located on adipocyte membranes can cause lipolysis.[21]

LIPO-102 and LIPO-202

Under investigation is an injectable form of the asthma medication ADVAIR® (salmeterol xinafoate with fluticasone propionate), known as LIPO-102 (Lithera Inc., San Diego, CA), for localized subcutaneous fat reduction via lipolysis. SX is a highly selective long-acting β_2-adrenergic receptor agonist, and fluticasone propionate (FP) is a synthetic trifluorinated glucocorticoid. Activation of β_2-adrenergic receptors located on human fat cells by salmeterol triggers the breakdown of triglycerides in these cells to free fatty acids and glycerol by lipolysis (Fig. 11.5). Glucocorticoids, such as fluticasone, have various effects on β-adrenergic receptor function in vivo: they enhance the coupling of β-adrenergic receptors to G proteins and the resulting activation of adenylate cyclase, and they decrease β-adrenergic receptor downregulation (tachyphylaxis) due to chronic receptor stimulation.

Overall, salmeterol stimulates lipolysis through activation of β_2-adrenergic receptors on fat cells and fluticasone upregulates the cellular pathways stimulated by salmeterol. In vitro studies confirm that SX liberates fat from human adipocytes in a manner similar to other β-adrenergic receptor agonists. Rat models, which lack β_2-adrenergic receptors, provided an early confirmation of the ability of the injection of SX to shrink fat pads (through other β-adrenergic receptors). Pig models, which provide the closest approximation to human fat, demonstrated that SX reduces fat layer thickness at doses up to approximately 1 µg; however, efficacy was reduced at higher doses due to tachyphylaxis. The glucocorticoid FP was found to enhance SX-induced lipolysis in in vitro and animal studies.

Patient selection

Pearl 3

Careful patient selection and setting realistic expectations are important for success with injectable fat-reducing therapies.

Pearl 4

Ideal patients should be nonobese and have localized areas of fat accumulation.

Patient selection and managing patient expectations are critical to all cosmetic procedures. Patients who are obese and seeking weight loss as a result of the treatment are not candidates for the treatment. The physician needs to emphasize that injectable therapies for fat loss *do not*

Figure 11.5 Receptor activity and mechanism of action of LIPO-202 (beta agonist, salmeterol xinafoate). *(Figure courtesy of Lithera Inc.)*

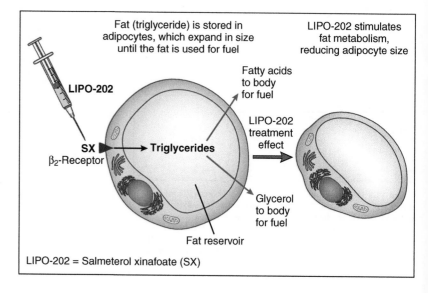

Fat (triglyceride) is stored in adipocytes, which expand in size until the fat is used for fuel

LIPO-202 stimulates fat metabolism, reducing adipocyte size

LIPO-202

Fatty acids to body for fuel

SX
β_2-Receptor

Triglycerides

LIPO-202 treatment effect

Glycerol to body for fuel

Fat reservoir

LIPO-202 = Salmeterol xinafoate (SX)

produce surgical outcomes, *will not* completely eliminate the localized fatty accumulation, and that therefore fat *may re-accumulate* with time and weight gain. Unlike submental liposuction (in the case of ATX-101) or abdominal liposuction (in the case of LIPO-202), which generate often dramatic, relatively immediate results, injectable treatments require multiple sessions over several months for clinically evident fat reduction. Additionally, while most patients demonstrate a treatment response, the severity of baseline fat volume generally determines how many treatments are necessary to yield an outcome that will be clinically meaningful to them.

Treatment

Pearl 5

Patients will require multiple treatments and will not have dramatic effects as with liposuction.

In clinical trials with LIPO-202, target patients were nonobese and had a BMI less than 30 (nonobese). The treatment area on the abdomen was mapped out prior to injection and a 30-gauge ½ inch needle was used without prior skin anesthesia. The treatment consisted of 20 abdominal injections for 8 consecutive weeks, with results seen in 1 month and peak results at 2 months. It is unknown at this time whether additional treatments will be needed for maintenance of fat-reducing effects.

In the ATX-101 clinical trials, injections were administered on a predefined grid placed on the submental ('under the chin') skin. Injections extended into the subcutaneous, preplatysmal plane using a 30-gauge needle. Ice immediately prior to and after treatment is generally suggested. Treatments are separated by 4 weeks apart and total three to six, depending on patient response. Persistence of effect has been observed as far out at 5 years in a majority of patients.

Outcomes

LIPO-102 and LIPO-202

Pearl 6

In the LIPO-202 clinical trials, the 0.4 µg SX dose demonstrated an average mean abdominal circumference reduction of 1.6 cm after patients received 20 weekly injections for 8 weeks.

Salmeterol xinafoate (SX) has been delivered to the anterior abdomen by subcutaneous injection in approximately 800 patients in six clinical studies conducted by Lithera; four of those studies were of the combination (LIPO-102), one study included both the combination (LIPO-102) and SX alone (LIPO-202), and the largest and most recent study (LIPO-202-CL-16) included only SX alone (LIPO-202). Each of these studies has provided preliminary evidence of efficacy in treating central abdominal bulging in nonobese patients through a variety of physical (e.g. laser-guided tape measurement) and clinical outcome (e.g. patient-reported outcome and clinician-reported outcome) endpoints.

In an early Phase 2 study, the most effective dose of SX (as part of LIPO-102, in combination with 1.0 µg FP) at reducing circumference was 0.5 µg injected subcutaneously once weekly for 4 weeks into anterior abdominal fat. Higher and/or more frequent dosing of SX (e.g. total weekly doses from 5.0 to 20 µg SX in combination with 1.0 µg FP) produced smaller reductions in abdominal circumference. These findings are consistent with the concept of tachyphylaxis (receptor desensitization and/or downregulation) often observed with β-adrenergic receptor agonists. In larger Phase 2b studies, peak reductions in abdominal circumference and volume, as well as improvements in subjective outcome measures, have been demonstrated with total weekly doses of SX between 0.4 and 1.0 µg (administered in combination with approximately 20 µg FP as 20–22 weekly 1 mL SC injections spaced 4 cm apart to the anterior abdomen for 8 weeks), with higher doses of SX (e.g. 10 µg) again being less effective. Each of these Phase 2 studies has demonstrated that reductions in abdominal bulging are related to the dose of SX (in the presence of a fixed dose of FP). A recently completed Phase 2 study confirmed the importance of SX alone to the SX + FP combination. Consistent with its mechanism of action, SX alone was responsible for 66–100% of the objective and subjective efficacy of the SX + FP combination.

Based on the sum total of in vitro animal and clinical data gathered to date, Lithera then decided to proceed with the development of SX alone (LIPO-202). LIPO-202 (SX for injection) was evaluated recently in the 513-patient, multicenter Phase 2 RESET Trial. One objective of this study was to evaluate the safety and efficacy of three doses of LIPO-202 (0.4, 1.0 or 4.0 µg total weekly dose) compared to placebo (0.9% saline) administered as 20 1 mL abdominal SC injections once per week for 8 weeks. Another objective was to evaluate the clinical utility of novel endpoints developed to measure changes in central abdominal bulging, including a Patient and Clinician Global Abdominal Perception Scale (P-GAPS, C-GAPS), a Patient and Clinician Photonumeric Scale (PPnS, CPnS), as well as the objective measurement of abdominal circumference and volume by a standardized laser-guided tape measure procedure and by MRI. Subjects were randomized to four treatment groups: placebo or three different doses of LIPO-202 (4.0 µg SX, 1.0 µg SX or 0.4 µg SX total weekly dose). The subjects received 20 SC injections weekly in the anterior abdomen for 8 weeks.

Significant (p < 0.05) increases in composite patient and clinician rating scale responders were observed with the optimal dose of LIPO-202 (0.4 µg) compared to

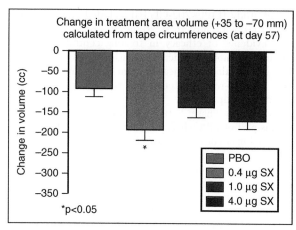

Figure 11.6 Significant reductions in mean abdominal circumference and volume assessed by laser-guided tape measure were observed with LIPO-202 (optimal dose, 0.4 µg) compared to placebo (PBO) (−1.6 cm/−192 cc vs −0.7 cm/−90 cc). *(Figure courtesy of Lithera Inc.)*

placebo. Significant reductions in mean abdominal circumference and volume assessed by laser-guided tape measure were observed with LIPO-202 (0.4 µg) compared to placebo (−1.6 cm/−192 cc vs −0.7 cm/−90 cc) (Fig. 11.6). Treatment effects were enhanced relative to baseline and to placebo in patients that remained weight neutral or lost weight compared to patients who gained weight (e.g. −2.7 cm vs −0.3 cm in mean umbilical circumference for 0.4 µg LIPO-202). Reduction in abdominal bulging was associated with significant increases in patient satisfaction. LIPO-202 produced clinically meaningful reductions in central abdominal bulging and may offer a novel, minimally invasive, nonablative approach to localized fat reduction.

ATX-101

Pearl 7

In the ATX-101 clinical trials, a 2 mg/cm^2 dose given in 4-week treatment intervals demonstrated greater than 1 grade improvement in submental fat in approximately 80% of patients 12 weeks after the last treatment.

In the Phase 2b randomized, double-blind, placebo-controlled, dose-ranging study, ATX-101 was well tolerated and demonstrated statistically significant efficacy as compared with placebo. The study enrolled a total of 129 subjects and was conducted in 10 dermatology and plastic surgery centers in the US. Multiple clinician and patient endpoints were assessed, as well as MRI to objectively quantify fat reduction. The study tested two drug-dosing regimens (1 and 2 mg/cm^2). Patients were divided into three groups: placebo, ATX-101 (1 mg/cm^2), ATX-101 (2 mg/cm^2). The patients received up to six treatment visits spaced at least 28 days apart. The mean number of

treatments for each group was as follows: 5.9 treatments for the placebo group, 5.3 treatments for the 1 mg/cm^2 group, and 4.9 treatments for the 2 mg/cm^2 group. At each treatment visit, up to 10 mL was administered at 0.2 mL/injection. The mean dose received per treatment was 6.02 mL for the placebo group, 5.62 mL for the 1 mg/cm^2 group, and 5.24 mL for the 2 mg/cm^2 group.

ATX-101 demonstrated statistically significant (p < 0.05) reductions in submental fat as compared with placebo as assessed by all measures: a validated clinician scale, patient-reported outcome scale, and magnetic resonance imaging (MRI) measurement for both fat volume and thickness. A statistically significant difference versus placebo was also shown on other patient-reported outcome measures, including instruments measuring subject satisfaction, patient impact, and chin attractiveness.

The Phase III trials for ATX-101, REFINE-1 and REFINE-2 compared the safety and efficacy of a 2 mg/cm^2 dose versus placebo for the reduction of submental fat.[22] The treatments were 4 weeks apart. Patients enrolled in the study had moderate to severe submental fat at baseline as determined through both validated clinician and patient-rating scales. The two primary efficacy endpoints of the trial were: 1) proportion of patients with a simultaneous improvement of at least one grade from baseline on the Clinician-Reported Submental Fat Rating Scale (CR-SMFRS) and the Patient-Reported Submental Fat Rating Scale (PR-SMFRS); and 2) proportion of patients with a simultaneous improvement of at least two grades from baseline on the CR-SMFRS and the PR-SMFRS. Secondary endpoints in the study included the reduction in volume of the submental region as measured using MRI, and the improvement in the appearance-related impacts of submental fat. The REFINE-1 and REFINE-2 trials demonstrated that ATX-101 was well tolerated by subjects. The physician ratings demonstrated that 79.5% of REFINE-1 and 78.3% of REFINE-2 subjects showed an improvement of at least one grade using the CR-SMFRS assessed 12 weeks after the last treatment. The patient ratings showed similar results with 82.4% of REFINE-1 and 78.9% of REFINE-2 subjects reporting at least a one grade improvement on the PR-SMFRS at 12 weeks after the last treatment.

The patient satisfaction data demonstrated that 88.9% of REFINE-1 and 84.2% of REFINE-2 ATX-101 treated subjects reported satisfaction with the treatment. The most common adverse events included swelling, pain, bruising, numbness and redness, and these were predominantly transient. It will be exciting to see more to come with this new therapy.

Complications and adverse events

Pearl 8

The two new agents appear to have excellent safety profiles with mild and transient adverse effects.

In LIPO-102 and LIPO-202 studies, there were no significant hematologic or cardiovascular adverse effects. There were no reports of atrophy, pigmentation, nodularity, or necrosis. The adverse events reported in the LIPO-102 studies included injection site bruising, erythema, hemorrhage, pain, and pruritus. Interestingly, there was minimal difference in injection site edema, erythema, irritation or any other local injection site reactions between LIPO-102 and placebo. The injection site reactions were mild and transient (and not different from placebo), greater than 95% rated them as mild, and there were no reports of severe reactions. In the LIPO-202 studies, safety was equivalent to placebo including injection site hematoma, pain, and erythema.

Pearl 9

In the LIPO-202 studies, the safety was equivalent to placebo, including injection site hematoma, pain, and erythema.

In REFINE-1 and REFINE-2 for ATX-101, there were no treatment-related serious adverse events. Less than 4% of subjects discontinued the study due to adverse events. The adverse events were predominately mild to moderate and include numbness (34.5% in REFINE-1, 33% in REFINE-2), edema (9%, 7.8%), bruising (9%, 8%), and pain (8%, 4%). Less common adverse events included erythema, induration, pruritus, paresthesia, and nodule formation.

These safety profiles of ATX-101 and LIPO-202 are consistent with their mechanisms of action, ablation and lipolysis, respectively. However, overall, the two new agents appear to have no long-term safety concerns.

Pearl 10

In the ATX-101 studies, adverse events were predominately mild to moderate and include numbness, edema, bruising, and pain.

Pearl 11

Less common adverse events for ATX-101 included erythema, induration, pruritus, paresthesia, and nodule formation.

Contraindications

Patients who are under 18 years of age should not receive this treatment. Obese patients are not candidates for the treatment and should be advised that this is for small, localized areas of fat. Pregnant and breastfeeding women also should not be treated. It is suggested that women wait at least 6 weeks after they have completed lactating prior to starting treatments.

Conclusion

A safe and effective injectable agent capable of reducing fat should become available in the near future, pending favorable review of clinical trial and pre-clinical data by regulatory agencies in the US and EU. As with other noninvasive methods, injectable methods aimed at reducing adipose tissue are not a replacement for liposuction, but, rather, another option for patients who desire a minimally invasive (nonsurgical) approach to reducing small collections of fat. Once in clinical use, a new arena within aesthetic medicine will broaden, opening opportunities for further investigation and development.

References

1. Jalian HR, Avram M. Body contouring: the skinny on noninvasive fat removal. Semin Cutan Med Surg 2012; 31(2):121–5.
2. Nelson AA, Wasserman D, Avram MM. Cryolipolysis for reduction of excess adipose tissue. Semin Cutan Med Surg 2009;28(4):244–9.
3. Nestor MS, Zarraga MB, Park H. Effect of 635 nm low-level laser therapy on upper arm circumference reduction: a double-blind, randomized, sham-controlled trial. J Clin Aesthet Dermatol 2012;5(2):42–8.
4. Ascher B. Safety and efficacy of UltraShape Contour I treatments to improve the appearance of body contours: multiple treatments in shorter intervals. Aesthetic Surg J 2010;30(2):217–24.
5. Jewell ML, Baxter RA, Cox SE, et al. Randomized sham-controlled trial to evaluate the safety and effectiveness of a high-intensity focused ultrasound device for noninvasive body sculpting. Plast Reconstr Surg 2011;128(1):253–62.
6. Rittes PG. The use of phosphatidylcholine for correction of lower lid bulging due to prominent fat pads. Dermatol Surg 2001;27:391–2.
7. Motolese P. Phospholipids do not have lipolytic activity. A critical review. J Cosmet Laser Ther 2008;10:114–18.
8. Duncan DI, Hasengschwandtner F. Lipodissolve for subcutaneous fat reduction and skin retraction. Aesthetic Surg J 2005;25:530–54.
9. Rotunda AM, Suzuki H, Moy RL, et al. Detergent effects of sodium deoxycholate are a major feature of an injectable phosphatidylcholine formulation used for localized fat dissolution. Dermatol Surg 2004;30:1001–8.
10. Gupta A, Lobocki C, Singh S, et al. Actions and comparative efficacy of phosphatidylcholine formulation and isolated sodium deoxycholate for different cell types. Aesthetic Plast Surg 2009;33:346–52.
11. Klein SM, Schreml S, Nerlich M, Prantl L. In vitro studies investigating the effect of subcutaneous phosphatidylcholine injections in the 3T3-L1 adipocyte model: lipolysis or lipid dissolution? Plast Reconstr Surg 2009;124:419–27.
12. Rotunda AM, Jones DH. HIV-associated lipohypertrophy (buccal fat-pad lipoma-like lesions) reduced with subcutaneously injected sodium deoxycholate. Dermatol Surg 2010;36:1348–54.
13. Rotunda AM, Kolodney MS. Mesotherapy and phosphatidylcholine injections: historical clarification and review. Dermatol Surg 2006;32:465–80.
14. Rotunda AM, Weiss SR, Rivkin LS. Randomized double-blind clinical trial of subcutaneously injected deoxycholate versus a phosphatidylcholine-deoxycholate combination for the reduction of submental fat. Dermatol Surg 2009;35:792–803.

15. Goldman MP. Sodium tetradecyl sulfate for sclerotherapy treatment of veins: is compounding pharmacy solution safe? Dermatol Surg 2004;30:1454–6.

16. Rotunda AM, Ablon G, Kolodney MS. Lipomas treated with subcutaneous deoxycholate injections. J Am Acad Dermatol 2005;53:973–8.

17. Odo YME, Cuce LC, Odo LM, et al. Action of sodium deoxycholate on subcutaneous human tissue: Local and systemic effects. Dermatol Surg 2007;33:178–88.

18. Thuangtong R, Bentow JJ, Knopp K, et al. Tissue-selective effects of injected deoxycholate. Dermatol Surg 2010;36:899–908.

19. Ellmerer M, Schaupp L, Brunner GA, et al. Measurement of interstitial albumin in human skeletal muscle and adipose tissue by open-flow microperfusion. Am J Physiol Endocrinol Metab 2000;278:E352–6.

20. Rotunda AM. Injectable treatments for adipose tissue: terminology, mechanism, and tissue interaction. Lasers Surg Med 2009;41(10):714–20.

21. Motolese P. Phospholipids do not have lipolytic activity. A critical review. J Cosmet Laser Ther 2008;10:114–18.

22. Carruthers J. REFINE-1 and REFINE-2: pivotal U.S. and Canadian Phase III Studies with ATX-101, an injectable drug for the reduction of submental fat. Presented at the American Society for Dermatologic Surgery (ASDS) Annual Meeting in Chicago, IL, October 5, 2013.

Cellulite: Anatomy, Etiology, Treatment Indications

12

Misbah Khan, Diana Bolotin, Nazanin Saedi

Key Messages

- Cellulite is an architectural condition of human adipose tissue
- Cellulite is characterized by a padded and nodular appearance of the skin in cellulite-prone areas, such as posterolateral thighs and buttocks in post-pubertal females
- Fundamental knowledge regarding its pathophysiology is lacking, which makes understanding and treating this condition a challenge

Introduction

Cellulite is thought of as a localized metabolic phenomenon that evokes an alteration in the female body silhouette. It presents a modification of skin topography evident by skin dimpling and nodularity that occurs mainly in women on the pelvic region, lower limbs, and abdomen. The change in skin topography is caused by herniation of subcutaneous fat within fibrous connective tissue leading to a padded or orange peel-like appearance (Fig. 12.1). Given the fact that the occurrence of cellulite is nearly universal in post-pubertal females, it can be thought of as a female secondary sex characteristic.

Cellulite is different from obesity and can be seen in women in all ranges of body mass index (BMI). Obesity is characterized by hypertrophy and hyperplasia of the adipose tissue that is not necessarily limited to the pelvis, thighs or abdominal areas. In contrast, cellulite is most commonly found in the, but not limited to, buttocks, thighs, and abdominal areas. It is a result of several ultrastructural, inflammatory, histochemical, morphologic and biochemical changes that produce the padded and orange-peel appearance of the skin.[1-3] Although there is no morbidity or mortality associated with cellulite, it remains a common cause of embarrassment to even the most physically fit women.

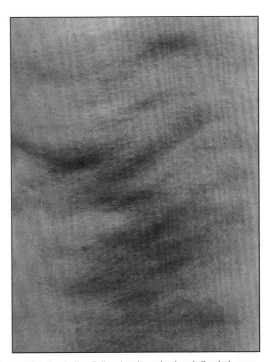

Figure 12.1 Grade II cellulite showing raised and dimpled areas while standing

Multifactorial etiologies of cellulite

Genetic predisposition plays a major role in the development of cellulite. The following factors are also important:

1. Gender differences – cellulite in its classic patterns affects women exclusively
2. Ethnicity – white women are more prone to cellulite than Asian women
3. Lifestyle – a diet excessively high in carbohydrates provokes hyperinsulinemia and promotes lipogenesis, leading to an increase in total body fat content, thereby enhancing cellulite

4. Sedentary lifestyle – prolonged periods of sitting or standing may impede normal blood flow, leading to more stasis and causing alterations in the microcirculation of cellulite prone areas

5. Pregnancy, as it is associated with an increase in certain hormones, such as prolactin, estrogen, progesterone and insulin and increased overall fluid volume – all of these factors promote cellulite lipogenesis and fluid retention.[4]

Anatomy and etiology of cellulite

Connective tissue alterations in cellulite anatomy

Cellulite is characterized by the presence of fatty protrusions through the dermohypodermal junction. A study by Rosenbaum et al.[4] reported similar findings using ultrasonography and full thickness wedge biopsy of the thighs under local anesthesia. Gross ex vivo and in vivo examination of the thighs showed a diffuse pattern of extrusion of underlying adipose tissue into the reticular dermis in affected (but not unaffected) individuals, directly correlating with clinical findings, such as dimpling and orange peel texture of thigh skin.

However, Pierard et al.[5] found no correlation in their study between the extent of these protrusions and clinical evidence of cellulite. In a study using autopsy specimens of 24 previously healthy women between 28 and 39 years of age with cellulite and 11 men and four women without cellulite, the authors revealed important distinguishing characteristics within the microarchitecture of subcutaneous connective tissue below the dermal–subcutaneous interface. They showed the presence of papillae adiposae rising into the 'pits and dells' on the undersurface of the dermis with sweat glands encased within. They found no correlation between the extent of this finding and the clinical type and severity of cellulite in women. In addition, the most distinguishing feature between cellulite-prone skin and unaffected skin was found to be uneven thickness of connective tissue septa, showing a few α-actin positive myofibroblasts in thicker strands. This finding correlated with the mattress phenomenon as seen on pinching of the skin corresponding with the areas where the septa are thicker and contain myofibroblasts. At the site of the skin dimpling at rest, the authors reported 'lumpy and loose' swellings interposed between thinner portions of the septa. Collagen fibers formed a delicate meshwork that was reminiscent of striae distensea. Acid proteoglycans and α₂-macroglobulin were abundant at these sites.

> **Pearl 1**
>
> Skin dimpling in cellulite and dermal stretch marks or so-called 'striae' may be similar conditions, with forces of distension acting in a perpendicular versus parallel fashion.

The study concluded that skin dimpling in cellulite and dermal stretch marks are similar conditions with forces of distension acting perpendicular versus parallel, respectively.[6] Hence, each can coexist in the same individual as is also commonly noted. They also found numerous blood vessels with an equal number of lymphatics (control vs

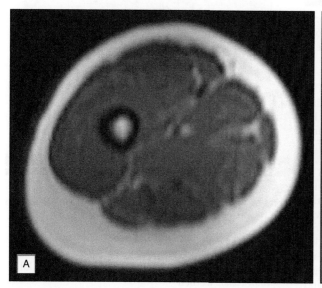 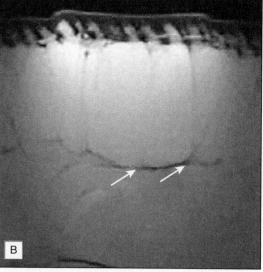

Figure 12.2 Magnetic resonance images of adipose tissue. **(A)** Hypodermis of the entire thigh that appears hyperintense. **(B)** High spatial resolution, two-dimensional image, 3 mm thick, of hypodermis on dorsal side of the thigh of a woman with cellulite. Camper fascia separates the adipose tissue into two layers. Fibrous tissue septa appear as thick, hypo-intense structures *(from Querleux B, Cornillon C, Jolivet O, Bittoun J. Anatomy and physiology of subcutaneous adipose tissue by in vivo magnetic resonance imaging and spectroscopy: relationships with sex and presence of cellulite. Skin Res Technol 2002; 8:118–24, with permission)*

affected) in the cellulite affected areas which is contrary to a popular belief that somehow cellulite prone areas have fewer lymphatics.

Pearl 2
Women with cellulite have a higher percentage of thinner, perpendicularly oriented hypodermal septa than unaffected women and men (Fig. 12.2).

Sexual dimorphism in cellulite skin architecture

The anatomic hypothesis of cellulite is based on gender-related differences in the structural characteristics of dermal and hypodermal architecture originally detailed by Nurnberger and Muller.[7] They described herniation of fat into the dermis, which is characteristic of female anatomy and which was later confirmed by ultrasound imaging as being low-density regions among denser dermal tissue.[4,8] Their study revealed that gender related differences are diffuse and not localized to the affected areas. They reported that dermal septa of the affected females are much thinner and more radially oriented than unaffected males, therefore facilitating the extrusion of adipose tissue into reticular dermis. In their study, cellulite-affected and unaffected female subjects both showed an irregular and discontinuous dermal–subcutaneous interface that was characterized by fat protrusion into dermis. The dermoadipose and connective tissue interface was smooth and continuous in male subjects.

Querleux et al.[9] revealed three principal orientations of the septa: perpendicular, parallel, and angulated at about 45° (Figs 12.3 and 12.4). Women with cellulite had a higher percentage of perpendicular septa than unaffected women (p < 0.001) or men (p < 0.01). For the other two directions, according to presence of cellulite, women with cellulite had a smaller percentage of septa

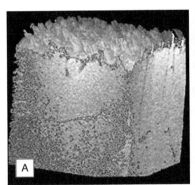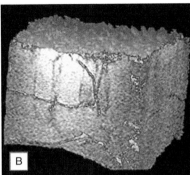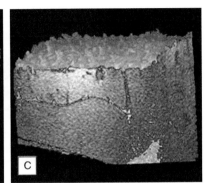

Figure 12.3 Visualization of three-dimensional topography of skin as seen by magnetic resonance imaging at the interface between the dermis and subcutaneous tissue. **(A)** Woman with cellulite. **(B)** Unaffected woman. **(C)** Unaffected male. Deep adipose indentations into the dermis are a hallmark of cellulite *(from Querleux B, Cornillon C, Jolivet O, Bittoun J. Anatomy and physiology of subcutaneous adipose tissue by in vivo magnetic resonance imaging and spectroscopy: relationships with sex and presence of cellulite. Skin Res Technol 2002; 8:118–24, with permission)*

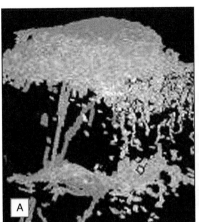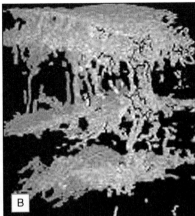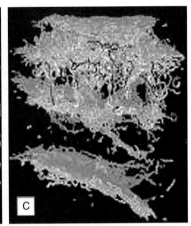

Figure 12.4 Visualization of the three-dimensional architecture of fibrous septa in subcutaneous adipose tissue as viewed by magnetic resonance imaging. **(A)** Woman with cellulite. **(B)** Unaffected woman. **(C)** Unaffected male *(from Querleux B, Cornillon C, Jolivet O, Bittoun J. Anatomy and physiology of subcutaneous adipose tissue by in vivo magnetic resonance imaging and spectroscopy: relationships with sex and presence of cellulite. Skin Res Technol 2002; 8:118–24, with permission)*

parallel to the skin (p < 0.001) and a higher percentage at 45° (p < 0.001).

Cellulite grading based on clinical severity

Cellulite can be divided into three main grades based on the clinical severity. Grade I is characterized by smooth skin without any dimpling upon standing and lying down, but the skin adopts a mattress-like configuration upon pinching, which forces fat into the reticular and papillary dermis. In grade II cellulite, a mattress-like appearance of cellulite is present upon standing but disappears with the patient in the supine position. Grade III cellulite can be seen in individuals who exhibit skin dimpling upon standing and can be exacerbated with pinching when they are in the supine position.[10] Although this classification has been used to identify various severity grades of cellulite, it does not take into account factors such as baseline skin laxity. Skin laxity may play a major role in the severity of cellulite despite clinically significant fat herniation. It is essential for the clinician to recognize all aspects of cellulite severity before considering a suitable treatment option.

Treatment of cellulite

A thorough medical history and a detailed physical examination are important parts of the treatment of cellulite. A history of bleeding disorders, vascular or lymphatic insufficiency, prior treatments for cellulite reduction including but not limited to skin tightening technologies, and surgeries, such as liposuction and body lifting procedures, must be taken into account. The medication history of prescription as well as over-the-counter drugs must be noted in the patient's records.

Physical examination is best performed with the patient standing upright wearing comfortable clothing. Any preexisting surgical scars, stretch marks and any obvious asymmetries should be noted and discussed with the patient at length. Tangential lighting may be used to determine the textural differences in various areas of cellulite-prone skin. Cellulite photography can be quite challenging. The color, angle, intensity and type of lighting may markedly affect the patient photographs in any given patient. It is therefore very important that baseline and follow-up photography is performed under standardized conditions of lighting, patient posture, baseline muscle tone (tightly flexed vs relaxed muscles), and underwear garments.

Pharmacological treatments

Catecholamines

> **Pearl 3**
>
> Several pharmacological agents available for the treatment of cellulite lack scientific evidence of long-term efficacy.

Numerous pharmacological agents are used to treat cellulite, including methylxanthines, retinoids, lactic acid, and herbal agents. Despite the plethora of topical treatments available at physicians' offices, pharmacies, spas, boutiques and over the internet, there is no large scale study showing the effectiveness of any of these therapies. Only two agents, aminophylline and retinoids, have been critically evaluated. Aminophylline stimulates β_2-adrenergic receptor activity and causes a localized lipolytic effect.[11]

> **Pearl 4**
>
> It is unlikely that topically applied pharmacological agents can alter the fundamental architectural alterations that exist in cellulite-prone areas.

Collis et al.[12] evaluated the effectiveness of topical aminophylline gel in combination with 10% glycolic acid and concluded that this therapy fails to improve cellulite. Although it has been hypothesized that topically applied aminophylline can penetrate through the dermis to cause significant lipolysis, this has not been scientifically proven. Additionally, the adrenergic receptors (AR) located in cellulite-prone areas are rich in α_2-ARs rather than β_2-ARs. Upon stimulation, α_2-ARs have an antilipolytic effect on lipid metabolism.[10] Nonetheless, these treatments are still used and patients report subjective improvement.

Retinoic acid

> **Pearl 5**
>
> Topically applied retinoic acid can improve skin collagen and may improve the skin texture in cellulite-prone areas.

Topically applied retinol 0.3% over a period of 6 months or more has been shown to improve cellulite.[13] These effects may be related to the known effects of retinoids (increasing dermal collagen thickness and improving the contours of elastic fibers). Studies have shown an increase in factor XIIIa-positive dendrocytes. Furthermore, retinol itself can act as an antiadipogenic agent by inhibiting the differentiation of human adipocyte precursor cells.

Peroxisome proliferator-activated receptors agonists

> **Pearl 6**
>
> Peroxisome proliferator-activated receptors are a recently discovered family of nuclear transcription factors that have been shown to enhance skin tightening and induce the uncoupling protein-1 on adipocytes.

Peroxisome proliferator-activated receptors (PPARs) are a newly discovered family of nuclear transcription factors with three receptor subtypes: PPAR-α, PPAR-β, and PPAR-γ.[14] PPARs bind to the peroxisome proliferator response element within the promoter region of the DNA in the target gene in the form of heterodimers with retinoid X receptor. All PPARs are found in adipocytes. Petroselinic acid and conjugated linoleic acid have been reported as potent PPAR-α activators, improving epidermal differentiation, reducing inflammation, increasing extracellular matrix components and eliciting skin tightening. They are also known to induce uncoupling protein-1 levels. Like retinoids, they also deliver pleotropic benefits. In vitro studies have shown that conjugated linoleic acid may prevent lipid accumulation in adipocytes.[4] Although promising, the efficacy of PPAR agonists in the treatment of cellulite is currently under investigation.

Unipolar and bipolar radiofrequency devices

Radiofrequency (RF) devices have recently gained supremacy in the treatment of cellulite as one of the most commonly performed nonsurgical treatments of cellulite. RF can be used to heat tissue at selected depths and volumes by changing the frequency, the configuration of the electrodes, and various other design features. The depth of penetration is inversely proportional to the frequency and those utilized range from 3 kHz to 24 GHz. The configuration of these devices may be either unipolar or bipolar. These devices include TriActive™ (Cynosure, Westford, MA) and VelaSmooth™ (Syneron Medical, Yokneam Illit, Israel). The purpose of integrating RF into cellulite treatment is to affect the connective tissue septa and fat lobules, both of which contribute to the appearance of cellulite. Of the available RF devices only VelaSmooth has been approved by the US Food and Drug Administration (FDA) specifically for the treatment of cellulite. The TriActive system combines a low-energy diode laser, contact cooling, suction and massage. This system has been shown to reduce cellulite.[14]

> **Pearl 7**
>
> Current unipolar and bipolar radiofrequency devices that are commonly employed for skin tightening can also be used to temporarily improve the skin laxity and dimpling associated with cellulite.

VelaSmooth combines infrared light (700–2000 nm) bipolar RF and suction with mechanical massage. Like VelaSmooth, the Alma Accent® RF system (Alma, Buffalo Grove, IL) and ThermaCool (Thermage, Hayward, CA) use RF and may be useful for the treatment of cellulite. Both Accent and ThermaCool are approved by the FDA for the treatment of wrinkles and rhytides. ThermaCool is a unipolar RF unit, while the Accent system is a combined unipolar and bipolar RF device. Of the two devices, only the Accent system has been evaluated for the treatment of cellulite.

> **Pearl 8**
>
> Radiofrequency devices are based on the principle of heat generation as a result of water and tissue interaction amongst adipocytes and dermal tissue.

The exact mechanism by which these platform devices work is yet to be elucidated. Bipolar RF devices are based on the principle of poor electrical conductance according to Ohm's law:

$$H = J^2\rho$$

where H = heat generated and ρ = tissue resistance.

The generated heat is strong enough to cause thermal damage to the surrounding adipose tissue and connective tissue septa (see Fig. 12.2). Bipolar RF devices may work at a depth of >3 mm and allow for better control and localized adipose tissue alteration. Unipolar devices use high frequency electromagnetic radiation (EMR). High frequency EMR induces high frequency rotational oscillations in water molecules which in turn produce heat (i.e. the greater the presence of water, the greater the tissue heat generation). The depth and breadth of thermal damage is greater and in a diffuse pattern, with less control than that provided by bipolar RF devices. In addition, low-energy lasers have wound healing properties, affecting endothelial cells, erythrocytes and collagen which potentially help in the healing of localized chronic inflammation still believed to be one of the major causes of cellulite.[11]

> **Pearl 9**
>
> Small studies with the currently available systems have shown mixed results.

A relatively recent study of VelaSmooth found a statistically significant decrease in thigh circumference at 4 weeks, but no immediate change or a persistent decrease at 8 weeks post-procedure.[15] Alvarez et al.[16] used animal models to reveal interesting results regarding the effects of RF treatment on dermal cellularity and collagen formation. The authors treated the backs of guinea pigs with RF in six sessions (one session/week) and took biopsy specimens after each session and at 2 months after the last treatment. They found a number of early changes in the papillary dermis such as expansion and edema due to vascular congestion. These changes were followed by an increase in cellularity and an accumulation of intercellular substances. Subsequently, an increase in collagen, elastic fibers and mucopolysaccharides was observed. These changes led to increased dermal thickness and collagen content. Although the animal model results clearly demonstrate increased dermal thickness, additional investigation is warranted.

Surgical treatments

Pearl 10

Surgical treatments for cellulite are based on localized lipo-sculpting, severing of the dermal septa that cause dimpling and skin tightening with laser lipolysis.

Liposuction and subcision

1. While liposuction may diminish fat deposits deep in the subcutaneous fat, its effect on the superficial components of fat as seen in cellulite can be disappointing
2. Skin necrosis can occur if liposuction is performed too superficially near the skin surface
3. Subcision can temporarily improve skin dimpling as seen in cellulite-prone areas
4. Long-term efficacy of subcision remains controversial.

Pearl 11

Liposuction and subcision may be performed safely under local anesthesia.

Liposuction if performed carefully at a deeper level under tumescent anesthesia may improve the bulges associated with cellulite. Subcision is a procedure that palliates skin dimpling by severing the septa that hold the herniated fat lobules. The procedure is performed under local anesthesia with a 16–18 gauge needle inserted into the subcutaneous fat in a direction parallel to the epidermis and the septa are sheared.[17] The results can be significantly enhanced if subcision is performed in conjunction with liposuction (Fig. 12.5). As herniated fat is close to the skin surface, if liposuction is performed too superficially it can potentially cause skin necrosis leading to worsening of the cellulite.

Laser lipolysis

Laser-induced lipolysis may reduce adipose tissue by causing thermal destruction of adipocytes and the surrounding collagen, thereby leading to a reduction in localized adiposities as well as a mild degree of skin tightening. The Nd:YAG laser has been used extensively for adipose tissue removal as well as for the treatment of cellulite. Kim and Geronemus[18] showed that there is an energy-dependent relationship with volume reduction during laser lipolysis using a 1064 nm Nd:YAG laser. They also demonstrated the release of subdermal bands of cellulite dimples thereby leading to a rather smooth skin surface after complete healing.

McBean and Katz evaluated the application of a sequentially firing 1064 and 1320 nm Nd:YAG laser device for lipolysis and skin tightening.[19] Their study revealed a 76–100% improvement in adiposities in 85% of the subjects and 51–75% improvement in 15% of the subjects. Histologic examination of the treated areas showed new collagen formation compared to baseline.

Cellulaze™ (Cynosure Inc., Westford, MA) is a laser that uses a 1440 nm Nd:YAG fiber with a novel delivery system to target the structural components of cellulite. The technology incorporates a unique side-light, side-firing fiber as well as a thermal sensing system for safer treatment. The system will stop firing the laser once the temperature inside the skin has reached 45–47 °C, which is enough to cause adipocyte deplaning, septal subcision and dermal heating.

DiBernado[20] reported that the use of the 1440 nm laser can reduce herniated fat in the dermis due to tissue coagulation leading to a 25% increase in skin thickness and a 29% decrease in skin laxity as seen by ultrasonography.

Figure 12.5 Treatment of cellulite using power-assisted liposuction and subcision. **(A)** Before and **(B)** 2 years after one treatment *(courtesy Dr. Khan, MH)*

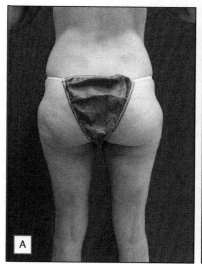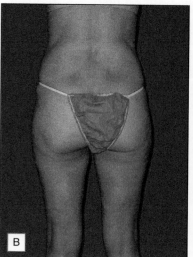

These results were maintained at 1-year follow-up visits as well. Although Cellulaze has shown good results for the treatment of cellulite, it is still a newer technology that requires additional studies performed at multiple centers in order to show a certain degree of predictability in terms of its outcomes regardless of the operator.

Pearl 12

Outcomes of such surgical procedures largely depend on the surgical techniques of the experienced surgeon.

Conclusion

Cellulite is an architectural disorder with multifactorial etiologies. Despite a large number of treatments available, all of which claim to work, few have proven significant lasting effects and many provide unpredictable results. The connective tissue septa that traverse and subdivide the hypodermis serve as suspenders that hold the adipose tissue. Theoretically, a procedure that will increase dermal thickness and reduce the volume of herniated adipose tissue in the hypodermis in a selective, predictable controlled and safe manner might clinically improve cellulite.[11]

References

1. Curri SB. Aspects morpho-histochimiques et biochimiques du tissue adipeux dans la dermohypodermose cellulitique. J Med Esth 1976;5:183–91.
2. Binazzi M, Grilli-Cicioloni E. A Proposito della cosidetta cellulite e della dermato-panniculopatia edemato fibrosclerotica. Ann It Derm Clin Sper 1977;31:121–5.
3. Ciporkin H, Paschol LH. Atualizaca terapeutica e fisiopatogenica da lipodistrofia ginoide (LGD) 'cellulite'. Sao Paulo, Brazil: Livraria Editora Santos; 1992.
4. Rosenbaum M, Prieto V, Rudolph L, Ship A. An exploratory investigation of the morphology and biochemistry of cellulite. Plast Reconstr Surg 1998;101:1934–9.
5. Pierard GE, Nizet JL, Pierard-Franchimont C. Cellulite: from standing fat herniation to hypodermal stretch marks. Am J Dermatopathol 2000;22:34–7.
6. Agache P, Ovid MT, Laurent R. Mechanical factors in striae distensae. In: Moretti GR, Rebora A, editors. Striae distensae. Milan: Symposium Publication Division Brocades; 1976. p. 87–96.
7. Nurnberger F, Muller G. So-called cellulite: an invented disease. J Dermatol Surg Oncol 1978;4:221–9.
8. Rosenbaum M, Prieto V, Rudolph L, Ship A. An exploratory investigation of the morphology and biochemistry of cellulite. Plast Reconstr Surg 1998;101:1934–9.
9. Querleux B, Cornillon C, Jolivet O, Bittoun J. Anatomy and physiology of subcutaneous adipose tissue by in vivo magnetic resonance imaging and spectroscopy: relationships with sex and presence of cellulite. Skin Res Technol 2002;8:118–24.
10. Khan MH, Victor F, Rao BK, Sadick NS. Treatment of cellulite. Part 1: pathophysiology. J Am Acad Dermatol 2010;62:361–70.
11. Khan MH, Victor F, Rao BK, Sadick NS. Treatment of cellulite. Part II: advances and controversies. J Am Acad Dermatol 2010;62:373–84.
12. Collis N, Elliot LA, Sharpe C, Sharpe DT. Cellulite treatment: a myth or reality: a prospective randomized controlled trial of two therapies, endermologie and aminophylline cream. Plast Reconstr Surg 1999;104:1110–14.
13. Kligman AM, Pagnoni A, Stoudmayer T. Topical retinol improves cellulite. J Dermatolog Treat 1999;10:119–25.
14. Boyce S, Pabby A, Brazzini B, Goldman MP. Clinical evaluation of a device for the treatment of cellulite: TriActive. Am J Cosmet Surg 2005;22:233–7.
15. Sadick N, Magro C. A study evaluating the safety and efficacy of VelaSmooth system in the treatment of cellulite. J Cosmet Laser Ther 2007;9:15–20.
16. Alvarez N, Ortiz L, Vicente V, et al. The effects of radiofrequency on skin: experimental study. Lasers Surg Med 2008;40:76–82.
17. Hexsel DM, Mazucco R. Subcision: a treatment for cellulite. Int J Dermatol 2000;39:539–44.
18. Kim H, Geronemus RG. Laser lipolysis using a novel 1064-nm Nd:YAG laser. Dermatol Surg 2006;32(2):241–8.
19. McBean JC, Katz BE. A pilot study of the efficacy of a 1064 and 1320-nm sequentially firing Nd:YAG laser device for lipolysis and skin tightening. Lasers Surg Med 2009;41(10):779–84.
20. DiBernado BE. Treatment of cellulite using a 1440-nm pulsed laser with one year follow-up. Aesthet Surg J 2011;31(3):328–41.

Massage/Mechanical Techniques: Cellulite Reduction

13

Sarah A. Malerich, Nils Krueger, Neil S. Sadick

Key Messages

- Cellulite is a multifactorial condition which benefits from a combination approach to treatment
- Reduced blood flow and lymphatic drainage, which worsen the appearance of cellulite, can be improved by mechanical manipulation
- Mechanical manipulation, while beneficial as a safe, noninvasive technique, does not result in the permanent resolution of cellulite

The etiology of cellulite has long been debated and several mechanisms have been proposed. While still controversial, understanding the pathophysiology behind cellulite is key when developing potential therapeutic treatments. This chapter will discuss mechanical techniques for the reduction of cellulite. To begin, it is important to underline the beneficial mechanism behind these types of treatment.

Several mechanisms exist leading to the hypothesized benefit of treatment with mechanical techniques. Cellulite is thought to be, in part, a kind of local edema due to water retained in the skin by an increase in glycosaminoglycans (GAG) in skin overlying cellulite areas, possibly due to estrogen-activated fibroblasts increasing GAG synthesis.[1] Increased GAG leads to an increased osmotic pressure and fluid retention. This is further aggravated by compressing small vessels, leading to reduced vascular flow and lymphatic drainage. Reduced blood flow along with compression of capillaries by adipocytes then leads to tissue hypoxia, local inflammation and increased collagen synthesis as well as inducing a local fibrotic response. This compression of capillaries by fat cells and arteriolar congestion was demonstrated in a photomicrograph of adipose tissue.[2] It has also been noted that activation of hypoxia-inducible factor, HIF1A, correlates with the appearance of collagen septa and that individuals with a rare mutant allele of this gene are protected from the development of cellulite.[1] Furthermore, cellulite has been associated with the presence of a specific polymorphism in the gene encoding angiotensin I converting enzyme, which then leads to increased angiotensin II formation resulting in reduced blood flow in the subcutaneous adipose tissue (SAT).[1]

In addition to reduced vascular and lymphatic flow, cellulite worsens with age as a result of thinning of the dermis. This suggests that increasing the thickness of the skin may lead to improvements in the appearance of cellulite.[3] Lastly, ultrasound shows herniation of fat into the dermis, identifying a possible benefit from treatments that result in SAT remodeling.[4]

Endermologie®

LPG® Endermologie® was developed by Louis Paul Guitay in 1970.[5] Originally used for the treatment of scar tissue and trauma, it was quickly realized that this device may also have a beneficial effect on the appearance of cellulite.[6] It has been cleared by the Food and Drug Administration (FDA) as a noninvasive massage system for the treatment of cellulite. This treatment works by creating positive pressure from rollers combined with negative pressure from aspiration influencing subcutaneous adipocytes. This mechanical strain is hypothesized to sublethally damage subcutaneous adipocytes, so they remodel with a better distribution of subcutaneous fat leading to an improved contour of the skin.

The Endermologie device consists of a treatment chamber with an aspiration system and two independent motorized rollers that roll and unroll skin folds. The treatment course consists of once- or twice-weekly treatment sessions lasting 10–45 minutes each. Wearing a special suit, which covers the patient's entire body except the face, neck, hands and feet, the patient lies in prone and supine positions as well as on their side to facilitate massage of the entire body.

In a study, 118 women aged 19–63 years underwent twice-weekly treatments for 15 total treatment sessions, each lasting 35–40 minutes.[5] Efficacy was graded using the Nürnberger–Müller scale (Table 13.1). By analyzing photographs of the hips and thighs before and after treatment, blinded dermatologists found a statistically significant improvement in cellulite. Of the 19 subjects starting with grade 3 cellulite, 63% improved to grade 2. Furthermore, 54% of the 51 subjects with grade 2 cellulite improved to grade 1. No improvements were detectable in patients beginning with grade 1 cellulite; however, only four subjects were graded at this level, and thus the sample size was very small. Overall, 53% of patients achieved a reduction in cellulite. Furthermore, 99% of subjects had an

Table 13.1 Nürnberger–Müller Scale

0	No or minimal alterations on skin
1	Orange peel appearance on the skin by pinch test or muscle contraction
2	Orange peel appearance at rest
3	Orange peel appearance at rest + raised areas and/or nodules

overall reduction in average body circumference suggesting an additional benefit from this device. Lastly, data from a subjective, questionnaire-based response demonstrated that only 4% of subjects were not satisfied with their cosmetic outcome, while 69% expressed high patient satisfaction. Patients were monitored for adverse effects at each visit and no irregularities, bruising, telangiectasia formation, dimples or other serious side effects were noted.

Based on the study results, this treatment seems to be a well-tolerated technique for temporarily reducing cellulite and body circumference and is best for moderate to severe cellulite. This technique is safe for all skin types, but should be avoided in anyone pregnant, with serious heart defects, or any type of malignancy.

Acoustic wave therapy

The acoustic wave therapy (AWT) system utilizes compressed air to form acoustic waves on target tissue. Pulses are generated by accelerating a projectile with pressurized air that strikes against a stationary surface, the vibration transmitter, generating acoustic waves, which propagate directly to target tissue. These waves are intended to stimulate metabolism and enhance circulation along with stimulating neovascularization and cell proliferation. Furthermore, collagen remodeling is stimulated within the dermis as a result of the increase in cell proliferation and release of growth factors.

The AWT device uses two transmitters. A high impact acoustic wave handpiece (C-ACTOR®) is used to increase cell wall permeability to enhance the release of triglycerides. The vibrating massage handpiece (D-ACTOR®) generates slow impact acoustic waves, stimulating the target tissue as well as enhancing blood and lymphatic flow. Before initiating treatment, a gel is applied to the skin to reduce energy loss and reduce friction as the device is moved across the skin. The high impact handpiece can be set at an energy level from 0.45 to 1.24 mJ/mm^2 depending on the sensitivity of the patient. The vibrating handpiece is set at an energy level of 1.4–5 bar. The handpiece is moved with slight pressure in contact with the skin towards lymph nodes and backwards without pressure in a centripetal direction.

In one study, 11 patients were treated once a week for a total of eight treatments to the thighs and buttocks versus a placebo group of six patients.[7] Assessments took place at baseline, before the last treatment and at 1 and 3 months following the last treatment. Measurement of efficacy was based on a patient questionnaire and both standard (two-dimensional) and three-dimensional photography. Out of the 11 treated patients, nine saw an improvement in the number and depth of dimples, eight visualized improvements in skin firmness and 10 noted improvements in skin texture. Standard photography was evaluated by blinded observers using the Modified Hexsel Scale which grades cellulite from 0 to 12. A statistically significant reduction in cellulite was assessed in the treatment group at 3 months following the last treatment, while no differences were identified in the placebo group. A study by Christ et al.[8] further evaluated cellulite reduction as well as improvements in skin elasticity. Participants were divided into two groups, one group receiving six treatment sessions over the course of 3 weeks and the other receiving eight treatment sessions over 4 weeks. Improvements in skin elasticity were seen in both groups, with a larger increase in the second group. This indicates that doing more treatments may have an additive effect to end results. Skin elasticity in the first group showed 45% and 75% increases at the 3- and 6-month follow-ups, respectively, whereas the second group had 95% and 105% improvements, at 3 and 6 months' post-treatment, respectively. Furthermore, based on ultrasound assessments, a change was detected in the collagen and elastin network within the dermis while the subcutaneous tissue became denser. These changes in elasticity are best seen in older individuals who already have poor elasticity. Adatto et al.[9] treated female patients with six treatments over 4 weeks, each receiving 3000 pulses. Follow-up appointments were conducted at 1 and 12 weeks following the last treatment. Consistent with the previous study, treatments resulted in statistically significant improvements in skin elasticity, as well as decreased depth of cellulite dimples. By the 12-week follow-up, further improvements were seen, indicating both a short and relatively long term effect.

AWT is a localized, noninvasive, and safe therapy. No major adverse effects were noted, although mild pain and reddening of the skin during treatment is a possible side effect. Redness generally self-resolves within a few hours. Continual improvement is noted for up to 3 months, indicating at least temporary results. Longer term follow-up studies are required to determine the length of efficacy and proper maintenance intervals as AWT is not a permanent solution. As outcomes were not affected by differences in demographic data, this seems to be an effective treatment for a diverse group of patients.

Combination therapy

VelaSmooth™

VelaSmooth™ is a noninvasive system, cleared by the FDA for improving cellulite. It combines infrared (IR) light (700–2000 nm wavelength), bipolar radiofrequency (RF), suction and massage. The combination of RF with optical energy reduces the amount of optical energy required for effective tissue heating and allows for the use of the device on most skin types as RF does not target pigment. Cellulite has a multifocal pathology and combination approaches have the ability to effectively treat different areas of involvement simultaneously. Within this device, RF targets the collagen septa, while IR and RF together induce dissociation of oxyhemoglobin, allowing oxygen to be available for fat metabolism.[6] Additionally, physical manipulation improves cellulite by increasing circulation and stretching connective tissue surrounding SAT. Altogether, this system may alter the architecture of fat protrusion and improve lipolysis.

Prior to treatment, the skin should be cleaned and a conductive lotion should be applied to moisturize the skin.[3] Lotion does not need to be reapplied during treatment unless it becomes difficult to move the applicator across the skin. It is important to make sure that the applicator is sealed to the skin throughout the treatment session and air being sucked into the applicator should not be audible. Each area should be treated for 5 minutes with three to six passes per area. The target endpoint is significant erythema and warmth, 40 °C to 42 °C, maintained for 5–10 minutes. Total treatment time is about 20–30 minutes for each side of the body. Treatments are recommended once a week for 4–6 weeks. The highest levels of IR light and RF energy should be used as tolerated by the patient; however, all treatment levels should never be set to their maximum parameters simultaneously. The range of treatment parameters available is listed in Table 13.2. The vacuum device should be set to a level of 1–2. In Fitzpatrick skin types IV–VI or in very tanned skin, IR light should be set to 1 or 2. If the patient does not experience lasting erythema or excessive heat, the level may be increased to 2 or 3.

Several studies have been conducted on this device (Table 13.3). Alster and Tanzi treated 20 patients with eight 30-minute sessions to the thighs and buttocks.[10] Patients received treatments twice a week for 4 weeks with assessments at 1, 3 and 6 months following the last treatment. Improvements in the appearance of cellulite were seen in 90% of patients, with a mean improvement of 50% at 1 month following the last treatment. Patients were satisfied with the treatment and all but one were interested in subsequent treatment to the control leg. Improvements were best at 1 month follow-up and still visible 6 months after the last treatment, indicating a need for ongoing treatment intervals to maintain results.

Kulick studied 16 patients who were also receiving twice-weekly treatments for 4 weeks. An RF energy of 20 W was used with 12.5 W of optical energy.[11] Follow-up assessments were conducted at 3 and 6 months following the last treatment. Mean improvements at 3 and 6 months' follow-up were 62% and 50%, respectively, as rated by the investigators. All patients graded their cellulite improvement to be greater than 25%.

Sadick and Magro also studied 16 patients, but for a slightly longer treatment period of twice-weekly treatments for 6 weeks on one leg with follow-up assessments at 4 and 8 weeks after the last treatment.[12] Maximum results were seen at the 4- and 8-week follow-up as assessed by an independent evaluator and the investigator.

Table 13.2 VelaSmooth™ treatment parameters

RF power	10–100 W
Optical power	10–100 W
Light spectrum	680–1500 nm
Vacuum level	150 mbar
RF	1 MHz

Table 13.3 Studies assessing the efficacy of the VelaSmooth™ device

Study	Treatment sessions	Treatment parameters	Treatment assessment	Overall cellulite improvement	Average improvement score
Alster & Tanzi	Twice weekly for 4 weeks	20 W RF 20 W IR	Quartile scale (similar to Sadick & Mulholland)	90%	1.82 at 1 month 1.4 at 3 mos 1.1 at 6 mos
Kulick	Twice weekly for 4 weeks	20 W RF 12.5 W IR	Investigator-graded	100%	62% at 3 months 50% at 6 months
Sadick & Magro	Twice weekly for 6 weeks	Variable	Investigator-evaluated Quartile-based scale	50% had >25% improvement	6% had >50% improvement at 4 weeks 25% had >50% improvement at 8 weeks
Sadick & Mulholland	Group 1: twice weekly for 4 weeks Group 2: twice weekly for 8 weeks	Max. 20 W RF Max. 20 W IR	Investigator-evaluated Quartile-based scale	100%	Group 1: 5% had >50% improvement at 4 weeks Group 2: 36% had >50% improvement at 4 weeks

Table 13.4 Initial treatment parameters for Triactive™

Fitzpatrick skin type	Power	Frequency	Duty cycle	Contact cooling	Treatment duration	Passes/zone
I–III	30 W	3 Hz	50%	10 °C	5 min/pass	3–5
IV–VI	20 W	3 Hz	50%	10 °C	5 min/pass	3–5

Sadick and Mulholland studied 35 female patients, 20 receiving biweekly treatments for 4 weeks and 15 receiving biweekly treatments for 8 weeks.[13] Patients were treated with 20 W RF energy and 20 W IR energy. All patients developed some improvement in cellulite, although higher levels of improvements were seen in patients that received 16 total treatments as opposed to 8 treatments, corresponding to a 50–75%, or a 75–100% improvement.

Possible adverse effects for this procedure include bruising, ranging from minor purpura to larger, diffuse bruising which self-resolved within 1 week. Other potential adverse events include erythema, pain, edema, bullae formation, scabbing, ecchymoses, post-inflammatory hyperpigmentation and scarring.[3]

Maximal effects are seen 4 weeks following the last treatment and, therefore, maintenance treatments at 4-week intervals may be indicated to maintain results.[6] This form of treatment does not result in permanent resolution of cellulite. Skin biopsies taken before and after treatment show no changes and the effects on cellulite remain unclear; however, clinical improvements are most likely to result from changes in subcutaneous or subfascial structures.[6]

Pearl 1

Monthly maintenance treatments are suggested after the original treatment series with the VelaSmooth™ device to maintain improvements.

Triactive™

Triactive™ is an FDA-cleared, noninvasive combination treatment consisting of a low-dose 810 nm diode laser, contact cooling, suction, and massage. This device is intended to reduce the appearance of cellulite by thickening the dermis, enhancing lymphatic and vascular flow by targeting endothelial cells as well as promoting neovascularization.[3,6] Meanwhile, rhythmic massage stretches the connective tissue, with the intention of smoothing the interface between the dermis and subcutaneous tissue.

This device offers the ability to adjust the depth and intensity of the rhythmic massage, which is controlled by frequency (0.1–5.0 Hz) and duty cycle (20–80%) settings[3]. Frequency is a measure of the number of aspirations per second and higher frequencies have a more superficial mechanism of action, while lower repetition stimulates deeper tissue. Higher duty cycles indicate

stronger action. Cooling may be adjusted from 10 °C to 25 °C. It is recommended to start at 30 W for Fitzpatrick skin types I–III and set the initial frequency at 3 Hz with a duty cycle of 60%. Frequency can eventually be increased to 4–5 Hz while decreasing the duty cycle to 50%. For darker skin types, Fitzpatrick skin types IV–VI, initial treatments are recommended to begin at 20 W and adjusted based on the level of discomfort and erythema. Contact cooling should always be kept at 10 °C (Table 13.4). The applicator should be sealed with no air being sucked into the chamber, promoting vacuum suction of the skin. Treatments last 5 minutes per treatment zone with 3–5 passes per zone for a total of 30 minutes of treatment time. At the end of treatment, there should be significant erythema of the skin and warmth radiating from the skin.

In one study, 19 patients were treated twice weekly for 6 weeks on one leg and compared with VelaSmooth treatments on the other leg.[6] A trend toward greater improvement was seen with TriActive, with a 25% average improvement versus 7% average improvement seen with VelaSmooth. However, these results were not statistically significant.

Gold[3] treated 10 women with 15 biweekly treatments. In all, nine patients completed the study and 50% improvement was seen in 80% of subjects based on a visual grading scale. Zerbinati et al.[14] treated 10 patients with 20-minute sessions three times per week. All patients noted an increase in skin tone and a reduction in the circumference of the treatment areas.

The only reported adverse effect was bruising which ranged from minor purpura to larger and more diffuse bruises which self-resolved within 1 week. When considering treatment approaches to cellulite, combination approaches offer potentially synergistic therapies directed at the multiple suggested pathophysiologies of cellulite.

SmoothShapes™

SmoothShapes™ is another device that is FDA-cleared for the short-term reduction of cellulite. It is a dual wavelength laser/suction device consisting of two rollers, a vacuum chamber, four 650 nm light-emitting diodes (LEDs, 1 W) and eight 915 nm laser diodes (15 W) in a 90 × 90 mm dimension. The 650 nm wavelength permeates the cell wall (Fig. 13.1) potentially allowing for the release of heated lipids which are then drained via the lymphatic system. This wavelength is minimally absorbed by the epidermal and dermal layers, allowing for enhanced penetration of subcutaneous tissue. Vacuum and roller

Table 13.5 Cellulite severity scale

Grade	0	1	2	3
Number of depressions	None	1–4	5–9	10+
Depth of depressions	None	Superficial	Medium depth	Deep
Morphological appearance of skin surface	No raised areas	'Orange peel'	'Cottage cheese'	'Mattress'
Grade of laxity	None	Slight	Moderate	Severe
Classification scale by Nürnberger & Müller	Zero grade	1st grade	2nd grade	3rd grade

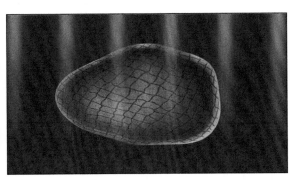

Figure 13.1 Modification of adipocyte permeation with 650 nm laser

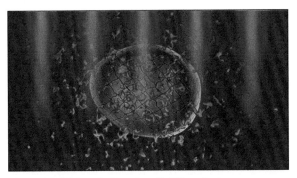

Figure 13.2 Heating of adipocytes with 920 nm laser

handpieces stimulate the lymphatic system through massage, reducing edema by increasing circulation. Meanwhile, the 915 nm wavelength causes a thermal effect within the adipocytes and increases the temperature slightly (Fig. 13.2). It further stimulates neocollagenesis and may improve lymphatic and vascular circulation.

The standard protocol for treatment is 10 minutes per area for eight biweekly treatments resulting in 80 minutes of total treatment time per treatment area. Suction should not exceed 500 mbar (375 mmHg). The technique should consist of linear movements of the handpiece following the direction of lymphatic drainage.

Lach[15] treated 102 female patients with an average of 14.3 treatments over 4–6 weeks. Up to 20 treatments were given with an average of three treatments adminis-tered every 2 weeks. Improvements in cellulite were seen based on before and after photos with no grading scale or quantification of improvement.

Kulick[16] treated 17 patients twice weekly for 6 weeks with follow-up assessments at 1, 3 and 6 months following the last treatment. Of the treated patients, 82% showed improvement at 1 month and 76% had improvement at both 3 and 6 months' follow-up based on physician-rated improvement. Based on participant surveys, 94% of patients felt their cellulite had improved. In addition, three-dimensional photography showed improved texture and a reduction in surface bulges.

Hexsel and colleagues[17] treated 15 female subjects with mild to moderate cellulite based on the cellulite severity scale (Table 13.5) with three treatments each lasting 30 minutes for 3 consecutive days, resulting in a total treatment time of 90 minutes. Follow-up assessments were performed at 7, 30 and 60 days post-treatment. At 60 days post-procedure, improvements were seen in at least one out of four categories in 14 subjects. Improvements in the number and depth of depressions were seen in 60% of subjects. It is noteworthy that 93% of patients reported they would get the treatment again and 71% felt that the treatment had improved their cellulite.

Lastly, Fournier et al.[18] treated 30 female patients with skin types I–V and mild to moderate cellulite of the thighs with 8 to 12 biweekly treatments. A high level of patient satisfaction was reported.

Most studies of this device reported no treatment related adverse events; however, possible adverse events include ecchymoses, erythema, edema, pain, burns, abrasions, scaling, infection, dyspigmentation and scarring.[3] SmoothShapes may be beneficial for short-term results, and, like other treatment options, requires longer follow-up studies to determine appropriate maintenance treatment intervals. Similar to other options for the mechanical treatment of cellulite, this device is an appropriate treatment option for average weight females with a normal BMI suffering from mild to moderate cellulite.

VelaShape™

VelaShape™ is cleared by the FDA for the temporary reduction of cellulite and circumferential reduction. It consists of broad-spectrum infrared light (700–2000 nm), bipolar RF, and vacuum suction pulses applied to the skin surface with a handheld applicator. VelaShape combines the previous VelaSmooth treatment head along with a smaller (30 × 30 mm) treatment head, known as the VelaContour. This newer version has 20% more power which allows for shorter treatment sessions as well as an improved interface terminal. VelaContour® may achieve up to 440 mbar of negative pressure, 20 W of peak IR energy and 23 W of peak RF energy. Meanwhile, Vela-Smooth may achieve up to 380 mbar of negative pressure, 35 W of IR energy and 60 W of RF energy.

VelaSmooth treatment sessions are recommended to be given biweekly over the course of 6 weeks with each session lasting 1 hour. VelaSpray Ease™ lotion is used to promote better performance. The application technique involves back and forth, circular, and zigzag movements to the treatment areas. The larger VelaSmooth applicator is used for large areas and is used for the majority of the treatment session while the VelaContour applicator is used for small curved areas and local fatty deposits.

A study of 11 females aged from 20 to 36 years assessed patients at baseline, after six treatment sessions, after the last treatment session and 4 weeks following the completion of treatment.[19] Based on clinical grading, significant improvements were seen on the buttocks, but no changes were observed on the thighs. Furthermore, significant reductions in hip circumference were seen, again with no changes in thigh circumference. All subjects noticed improvement and most of them considered it to be rapid in onset. A total of six subjects noticed improvements after 3 weeks of treatment and one subject did so after 2 weeks. Overall, patients were satisfied and would undergo the treatments again. Most patients in this study were of Fitzpatrick skin type III. One subject dropped out due to pain related to the first treatment.

No adverse effects have been reported and subsequent, larger studies are required in order to obtain more data regarding the safety and efficacy of this device. Furthermore, this device should be tested on diverse populations and skin types in order to select the appropriate patient population for its use.

Vibro Light™

Vibro Light™ is a low level laser therapy (LLLT) consisting of a 635 nm wavelength diode laser and vibration therapy. This device is believed to form transitory pores in adipocyte cell membranes leading to the collapse of adipocytes. LLLT is intended to stimulate mitochondria to produce adenosine triphosphate (ATP) leading to increased cyclic adenosine monophosphate (cAMP), which then leads to conversion of triglycerides to free fatty acids and glycerol that are able to pass through these transitory pores.[20] Meanwhile, vibration stimulates skeletal muscle potentially leading to improvements in endothelial function and increased local metabolism as well as improving vascular and lymphatic drainage. This treatment option

may be recommended for those patients who do not follow an exercise program and thus do not sufficiently stimulate their skeletal muscle on their own.

In one study, patients received biweekly treatments for 4 weeks with an oscillating platform at 5 Hz for 3 minutes, LLLT for 15 minutes, oscillating platform at 12 Hz in combination with LLLT for 5 minutes, and oscillating platform at 5 Hz in combination with LLLT for 5 minutes for a total time of 28 minutes.[19] Adipose tissue taken from an abdominoplasty specimen was examined histologically 7 days after the last treatment to this area. A reduction in fat thickness was demonstrated. Blood tests evaluated the safety of this procedure with no alteration in hepatic function markers and mild decreases in triglycerides and very-low density lipoproteins noted. No adverse effects, including paresthesias, hematomas, ecchymoses or edema, were reported.

Conclusions

Several devices are available that use massage or mechanical energy alone or in combination with other modalities to treat cellulite (Table 13.6). These devices have been evaluated in a variety of clinical studies and used in clinical practice. Although no mechanical device results in permanent resolution of cellulite, these treatment options offer patients a safe way to improve the appearance of their cellulite. These devices are best used for those individuals with a normal BMI and stable weight or as maintenance treatment after a minimally invasive procedure. It is important to educate patients as to the expected results and patients should understand the likely need for several treatment sessions as well as periodic maintenance sessions with these therapies.

Table 13.6 Brief overview of treatments discussed in this chapter

Device	Mechanism
Endermologie	Noninvasive massage system
Acoustic Wave Therapy	Generates acoustic waves against target tissue
VelaSmooth™	Combined IR light, bipolar RF, suction and massage
Triactive™	Combined low-dose diode laser, contact cooling, suction and massage
SmoothShapes™	Combined dual wavelength/laser suction device
VelaShape™	Combined broad-spectrum IR light, bipolar RF, and vacuum suction
Vibro Light™	Combined low level laser therapy and vibration

CASE STUDY 1

The patient is a 27-year-old female with mild to moderate cellulite on her upper thighs and buttocks (Fig. 13.3A). The patient requested a treatment to improve the appearance of her cellulite as well as a reduction of thigh circumference. The patient attended eight treatment sessions over 2 months (twice per week) of acoustic wave therapy. At each session, she received 2500 planar pulses per leg with 1.1 mJ/mm^2 and 4000 radial pulses with up to 4.0 bar. Two months after treatment the skin surface is smoothed out and the circumference of the thighs is distinctly reduced (Fig. 13.3B).

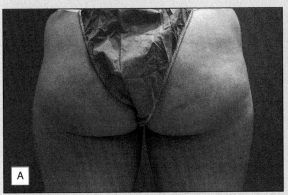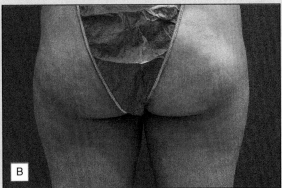

Figure 13.3 Case study 1. Acoustic wave therapy. **(A)** Before and **(B)** 2 months after treatment

CASE STUDY 2

A 35-year-old female presented with mild to moderate cellulite on her upper thighs and buttocks (Fig. 13.4A). Although exercising 3–5 times a week, the patient complained about resistant dimples and uneven skin topography. The patient attended eight treatment sessions (twice per week) of SmoothShapes therapy. The skin surface is even and dimples at the thighs have almost disappeared 2 weeks later (Fig. 13.4B). Some horizontal grooves on the buttocks are still apparent, but smoothed out.

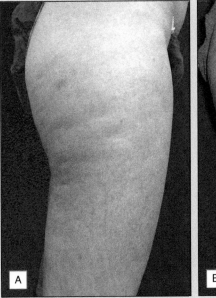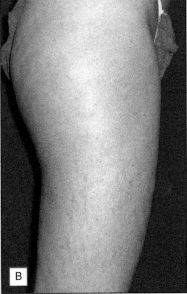

Figure 13.4 Case study 2. SmoothShapes therapy. **(A)** Before and **(B)** 2 weeks after 8 treatment sessions

References

1. Emanuele E. Cellulite: advances in treatment: facts and controversies. J Clin Dermatol 2013;31:725–30.

2. Omi T, Sato S, Kawana S. Ultrastructural assessment of cellulite morphology: clues to a therapeutic strategy. J Laser Ther 2013;22(2):131–6.

3. Gold M. The use of rhythmic suction massage, low level laser irradiation, and superficial cooling to effect changes in adipose tissue/cellulite. Lasers Surg Med 2006;38:65.

4. Salter DC, Hanley M, Tynan A, et al. In-vivo high definition ultrasound studies of subdermal fat lobules associated with cellulite. J Invest Dermatol 1990;29:272–4.

5. Kutlubay Z, Songur A, Engin B, et al. An alternative treatment modality for cellulite: LPG endermologie. J Cosmet Laser Ther 2013;15:266–70.

6. Wassef C, Rao BK. The science of cellulite treatment and its long-term effectiveness. J Cosmet Laser Ther 2012; 14:50–8.

7. Russe-Wilglingseder K, Russe E, Vester JC, et al. Placebo controlled prospectively randomized, double-blinded study for the investigation of the effectiveness and safety of the acoustic wave therapy (AWT®) for cellulite treatment. J Cosmet Laser Ther 2013;15:155–62.

8. Christ C, Brenke R, Sattler G, et al. Improvement in skin elasticity in the treatment of cellulite and connective tissue weakness by means of extracorporeal pulse activation therapy. J Aesth Surg 2008;28(5):538–44.

9. Adatto M, Adatto-Neilson R, Servant JJ, et al. Controlled, randomized study evaluating the effects of treating cellulite with AWT®/EPAT®. J Cosmet Laser Ther 2010;12:176–82.

10. Alster TS, Tanzi EL. Cellulite treatment using a novel combination radiofrequency, infrared light, and mechanical tissue manipulation device. J Cosmet Laser Ther 2005;7(2): 81–5.

11. Kulick M. Evaluation of the combination of radiofrequency, infrared energy and mechanical rollers with suction to improve skin surface irregularities (cellulite) in a limited treatment area. J Cosmet Laser Ther 2006;8(4):185–90.

12. Sadick N, Magro C. A study evaluating the safety and efficacy of the VelaSmooth system in the treatment of cellulite. J Cosmet Laser Ther 2007;9(1):15–20.

13. Sadick NS, Mulholland RS. A prospective clinical study to evaluate the efficacy and safety of cellulite treatment using the combination of optical and RF energies for subcutaneous tissue heating. J Cosmet Laser Ther 2004;6(4):187–90.

14. Zerbinati N, Rafaella V, Beltrami B. The Triactive system: a simple and efficacious way of combating cellulite. DEKA®; 2003, July.

15. Lach E. Reduction of subcutaneous fat and improvement in cellulite appearance by dual-wavelength, low level laser energy combined with vacuum and massage. J Cosmet Laser Ther 2008;10:202–9.

16. Kulick MI. Evaluation of a noninvasive, dual-wavelength laser-suction and massage device for the regional treatment of cellulite. Plast Reconstr Surg 2010;125(6):1788–96.

17. Hexsel D, Siega C, Schilling-Souza J, et al. Noninvasive treatment of cellulite utilizing an expedited treatment protocol with a dual wavelength laser-suction and massage device. J Cosmet Laser Ther 2013;15:65–9.

18. Fournier N, Pankratov M, Aubree AS, et al. Cellulite treatment with photomology technology. American Society for Laser Medicine and Surgery Meeting. National Harbor (MD), 5 January, 2009.

19. Hexsel DM, Siega C, Schilling-Souza J, et al. A bipolar radiofreqency, infrared, vacuum and mechanical massage device for treatment of cellulite: a pilot study. J Cosmet Laser Ther 2011;13:297–302.

20. Savoia A, Landi S, Vannini F, Baldi A. Low-level laser therapy and vibration therapy for the treatment of localized adiposity and fibrous cellulite. Dermatol Ther 2013;3:41–5.

Lasers and Lights: Cellulite Reduction

14

Stefanie Luebberding, Kathryn M. Kent,
Macrene Alexiades-Armenakas

Key Messages

- Laser and light-based modalities are one of the latest advances in the treatment of cellulite

- External light irradiation has the capacity to trigger a photobiomodulatory effect in the targeted tissue stimulating several cellular functions such as neocollagenesis or adipocyte lipolysis. The therapeutic benefit stems from a thermogenic or nonthermogenetic effect

- Green (532 nm), red (650 nm) and infrared (700–2000 nm) laser light in a low- or high-energy level is used for cellulite treatments

- Depending upon the wavelength, intensity, and total energy delivered, the therapeutic benefit of light-based treatment modalities stems from a thermogenic or nonthermogenetic effect

- Long-term effectiveness has not yet been proven with any of the medical devices available

Introduction

Cellulite is a topographic and localized alteration of the skin that creates a dimpled or 'orange peel' appearance, most commonly found on the posterolateral thighs, buttocks, and abdomen. In 1978, Nürnberger and Müller[1] first described cellulite as a result of sex-related differences in the structure of skin and subcutaneous tissue. The perpendicular orientation of the fibrous septa in women allows protrusion of the underlying fat, creating a rippled appearance. The oblique nature of these fibers in men appears to prevent this phenomenon. More recent studies confirm these sex-related structural differences,[2] and further explain the appearance of cellulite to be a result of the convergence of several overlapping physiological alterations such as focally enlarged fibrosclerotic septa that tether the skin in areas of cellulite, or an uneven dermal–hypodermal interface.[3,4]

Although precise epidemiological data are lacking, most studies claim that cellulite is present in over 80–90% of post-pubertal women.[3] Given the ubiquitous nature of cellulite, it is more appropriately thought of as a secondary sex characteristic rather than a disease. However, as digitally altered images of women's bodies in the media have become the new standard of 'beauty', the perception is that cellulite affects only the unlucky few. As such, it has become a major cosmetic concern for women.

Treatment

Although cellulite is not a disease in the proper sense and there is currently no cure for it, numerous treatment modalities have been developed to improve the appearance of cellulite. There are a myriad of over-the-counter creams that purport to remove cellulite; however, there is little evidence demonstrating efficacy of these products. Currently available medical devices aim to target the structural features of cellulite. In addition to the application of ultrasound and radiofrequency (RF) energy and mechanical manipulation and disruption, laser and light-based modalities are one of the latest advances in the treatment of cellulite.

Historically, various light sources have been used in physical therapy to reduce pain and inflammation, although the exact mechanism of action was widely unknown. Only recently, it became evident that external laser and light emitting diode (LED) irradiation has the capacity to trigger a photobiomodulatory effect in the targeted tissue stimulating several cellular functions such as neocollagenesis or adipocyte lipolysis. Depending on the wavelength, intensity, and total energy (J/cm^2) delivered, the therapeutic benefit may stem from a thermogenic or nonthermogenetic effect.[5,6]

VelaSmooth™

The VelaSmooth™ technology (Syneron Medical Ltd, Yokneam, Israel) is based on the simultaneous application of light energy to the tissue at a controlled infrared (IR) wavelength, conducted RF energy, and mechanical manipulations of the skin and fat layer.[7] It was the first medical light-based device to achieve FDA approval. Bipolar RF (up to 35 W) and infrared light in the wavelength range of 700–2000 nm are used to heat the subcutaneous tissue, while vacuum suction is applied to shape the skin for optimal delivery of RF energy up to a depth of 15 mm. Proposed tissue reaction to the VelaSmooth technology is an increase in local blood supply to the subcutaneous

Table 14.1 Overview of devices related to the VelaSmooth technology

	IR power	IR light spectrum	RF power	RF frequency	Vacuum suction	Massage
VelaSmooth™ Plus	Up to 35 W	700–2000 nm	Up to 35 W	1 MHz	200 mbar	Yes
VelaShape™ II	Up to 35 W	700–2000 nm	Up to 60 W	1 MHz	200 mbar	Yes
VelaShape™ III	Up to 3.3 W	850 nm	Up to 150 W	1 MHz	350 mbar	Yes

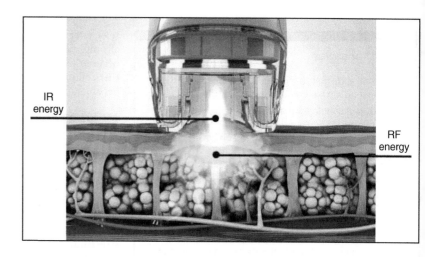

Figure 14.1 Schematic representation of the VelaShape™ III technology *(with permission of Syneron Medical Ltd, Yokneam, Israel)*

tissue promoting an increase in fat metabolism. Eventually, the mechanical action due to suction and massage lead to a collapse of fat cell clusters and fibrous bands smoothing the skin surface.[7]

Further advancements of the VelaSmooth technology are the VelaShape™ II and VelaShape III devices (see Table 14.1). Both use the combined modality treatment of controlled heating and mechanical action (Fig. 14.1), but offer a more powerful RF power up to 150 W allowing a faster and deeper heat penetration into the tissue.[8] With these alterations, treatment duration is shortened by approximately 30%, and fewer treatment sessions are needed.[9]

A conductive fluid is used immediately before treatment to hydrate the skin surface. Using the handheld applicator, the area of interest should be treated with 4–6 passes by moving the handpiece back and forth several times. Thereby, the applicator must be in full contact with the skin surface area to allow the vacuum to be most effective and to ensure that the electrode rollers are fully coupled to the skin. The endpoint of treatment is achieved when significant erythema and warmth radiating from the treated skin is observed. The average duration of a thigh and buttock treatment lasts about 30–45 minutes.[9,10] The treatment is generally very well tolerated with only minimal to no discomfort. However, heating sensations and pinching as well as transient erythema, bruising and localized swelling have been reported.[7,11,12]

One of the first studies evaluating the safety and efficacy of the VelaSmooth system was published by Sadick and Mulholland in 2004.[7] Thirty-five female subjects with cellulite and/or skin irregularities on the thighs and/or buttocks received twice-weekly treatments for 4 and 8 weeks. Circumferential measurement and pre- and post-treatment photographs were used to grade the level of improvement. In most of the patients the thigh area showed an overall mild to moderate improvement in skin smoothing and cellulite appearance. The overall mean decrease in thigh circumference was approximately 0.8 inches.

Similar results were assessed in a study conducted by Alster and Tanzi[11] who treated 20 female subjects with moderate bilateral thigh and buttock cellulite with eight biweekly treatments to a randomly selected side with the contralateral side serving as the control. Clinical improvement was scored from comparable photographs using a quartile grading scale by two blinded evaluators. Ninety percent of patients noticed overall improvement and clinical scores averaged 50% improvement upon completion of the study.

In another split side study, 10 subjects received biweekly treatments for 12 weeks to one side of the buttocks with the opposite side serving as the control. All patients were satisfied with the results 2 months post-treatment and requested treatment of the nontreated side. Histological analysis showed fiber compaction and

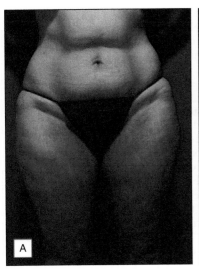 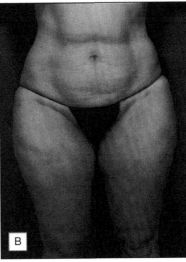

Figure 14.2 The abdomen treated with the VelaShape™ III at **(A)** baseline, and **(B)** following five treatments *(with permission of R. Amir, MD)*

tightening of skin layers, including the subcutis, which may account for the observed clinical improvement (Fig. 14.2).[12]

Long-term results for both the thigh and abdomen were first reported by Wanitphakdeedecha and Manuskiatti[10] 1 year post-treatment. The long-term evaluation suggests that most of the circumference reduction is maintained for at least 1 year after the completion of 8–9 treatments twice a week (6.23% after the final treatment, and 5.50% 1 year later).

> **Pearl 1**
>
> Baseline and follow-up standardized digital non-flash photographs with identical positioning and lighting are strongly recommended in order to track efficacy.

TriActive™

The TriActive™ (Cynosure Inc., Chelmsford, MA), a class II over-the-counter device, merges suction, massage, and contact cooling with the application of an 808 nm diode low-level laser.

Gold[13] treated 10 female subjects with a total of 15 biweekly treatments, utilizing protocols determined by the device manufacturer. Of the nine subjects completing the study, there was an overall change on the Visual Cellulite Grading Scale from 2.44 at baseline, to 1.44 post-treatment. This represented an approximately 50% improvement. Length of follow-up was not noted in this study. Boyce et al.[14] found an improvement of cellulite, skin texture, size and skin tone after biweekly treatments for 6 weeks. They stated that the greatest improvement was seen in those with the least symptoms.

In a study comparing the TriActive and the VelaSmooth devices, Nootheti et al. treated 26 female patients biweekly for 6 weeks. Treatment was randomized with use of the TriActive on one side and VelaSmooth on the other

side. Patients were evaluated with photographs and circumferential thigh measurements before treatment and after the final treatment. Both devices produced modest improvements in the appearance of cellulite and the average mean percent age change calculated was roughly the same for both treatments.[15]

Verjú

Verjú (Erchonia Corporation, McKinney, TX) is another low-level laser method that uses six 532 nm green diodes for improving the appearance of cellulite. Unlike common high-energy laser treatments, low-level laser therapy (LLLT) does not cause significant changes in the tissue structure, but, among its effects, it modulates adipocyte function by causing a transitory pore in the cell membrane, which purportedly drains the fat cell.

To date, only one study, by Jackson et al.[16] has been published on this device. This double blind, placebo-controlled randomized trial evaluated 68 subjects who received three weekly treatment sessions 2–3 days apart. During each session, the front and back of the hips, thighs, and waist were exposed for 30 minutes in total. All subjects in the LLLT group achieved a decrease of one or more stages on the Nürnberger–Müller grading scale and a significant decrease in thigh circumference at the 2-week study endpoint and 6-week follow-up evaluation. About 62.1% of the LLLT-treated subjects were 'very satisfied' or 'somewhat satisfied' with the clinical outcome.[13]

> **Pearl 2**
>
> More meaningful clinical outcomes from noninvasive modalities are obtained in patients with less severe cellulite grades.

SmoothShapes®

The SmoothShapes® (Cynosure Inc., Chelmsford, MA) also uses lower-level 915 nm continuous wave laser and

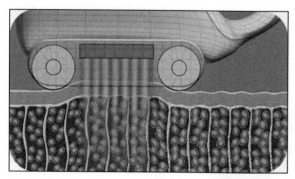

Figure 14.3 Schematic representation of the SmoothShapes® handheld roller *(with permission of Cynosure Inc., Chelmsford, MA)*

650 nm LED energy in combination with mechanical manipulation of the skin to treat cellulite (Fig. 14.3). This patented technology is called Photomology® and promises targeted treatment of adipose cells. The infrared 915 nm laser light is known to be among the peak absorption spectra for fat,[17] while the low-level 650 nm light improves cell membrane permeability due to the creation of temporary 'pores' allowing the fat to escape in the extracellular space.[5] Mechanical massage then helps in the movement of the fat into the lymphatic system and promotes lymphatic drainage, subcutaneous blood flow, new collagen deposition, as well as firming and toning of the skin.[5,18] A typical treatment session is about 20 minutes for a set of body parts. Thus far, no adverse events have been reported; however, transient side effects occur. Patients may experience pain or tingling during treatment, changes in urinary habits, swelling, and skin redness.[19,20]

In one of the first studies, using a prototype of the SmoothShapes device, Lach[20] compared the efficacy and safety of low-level, dual-wavelength laser energy and massage with massage alone for the reduction of subcutaneous fat and the improvement of cellulite. The thighs of 102 subjects were randomized to laser light plus massage, or to massage alone. A mean of 14.3 treatments were administered over a period of 4–6 weeks. Fat thickness was found to decrease by 1.19 cm^2 in the leg treated with laser and massage and increase by 3.82 cm^2 in the leg treated with massage alone as assessed with MRI. Overall, about 82.26% of the subjects responded to the treatment. A study by Gold et al.[19] confirmed these results and further shows that the upper thigh responded best to the treatment in comparison with the middle and lower thigh, with the maximum circumference reduction of −0.82 cm occurring at 1 month post-treatment.[20]

Kulick[21] treated 20 women with cellulite of the lower thighs with the SmoothShapes device 15 minutes per thigh biweekly for 4 weeks. Photographs were taken using standard photography as well as with VECTRA® three-dimensional photography. Analysis showed 82% improvement at 1 month and 76% improvement at 6 months post-treatment. About 75% of the subjects reported an improvement in cellulite irregularities such as dimples, and about 94% felt their contour improvements remained at 6-month follow-up.

Cellulaze™

Cellulaze™ (Cynosure Inc., Chelmsford, MA) is a minimally invasive modality approved for the treatment of cellulite. A pulsed 1440 nm Nd:YAG laser delivers energy to the dermal–hypodermal interface with the objective of treating structural features that cause the clinical appearance of cellulite. Firstly, the technology is believed to smooth the uneven dermal–hypodermal interface by selectively melting the hypodermal adipocytes that protrude into the dermis. Secondly, it should extract the hypodermal septa connecting the dermal and muscle layers by thermal subcision. Finally, the technique heats the dermis to increase skin thickness and elasticity by stimulating neocollagenesis and collagen remodeling.[22]

The Cellulaze system delivers laser energy directly to the subdermal tissue without penetrating the upper skin layer. The target area is therefore infused with tumescent solution to a maximum total volume of 1 liter, before a 600 μm 'side-firing' fiber enclosed in a 1 mm cannula is introduced through a small incision close to the target area below the skin surface. The Cellulaze procedure is then divided into three steps (Fig. 14.4). In the first phase, the cannula, moved in a fanning motion, is placed in the 'down' position in order to thermally denature hypodermal adipocytes, and this is followed by the 'horizontal' position that breaks the hypodermal septa by thermal subcision. In the last position, so called 'up', the fiber is positioned 2–3 mm below the skin surface to stimulate collagen remodeling, and to increase skin elasticity by heating the tissue. Both skin surface and subdermal temperature are monitored during the procedure to prevent thermal burns. Upon completion of the laser procedure, patients should wear a compression garment for up to 3 weeks post-treatment.[22] Generally, the Cellulaze procedure is relatively free of any side effects, but mild discomfort, bruising, swelling, itching, and numbness may occur. All side effects resolve within 3 months.[22,23]

In a study by DiBernardo[22] 10 female subjects with cellulite of the thighs received a single treatment with a 1440 nm pulsed laser to evaluate efficacy, safety, and duration of clinical benefit. At 1, 3, 6 and 12 months, treatment success was evaluated using two- and three-dimensional digital photography, suction chamber method, ultrasound, as well as subject and physician surveys using a five point scale (0, worse – 4, excellent). At 1 year, physician evaluation revealed mean scores of 3.4 for firmness, overall reduction, and overall improvement and 3.9 for skin texture. Patients rated overall reduction of cellulite as 3.2, skin texture improvement as 3.0 and overall satisfaction as 3.7 at 1 year. All patients achieved an increase in skin thickness and elasticity as compared to baseline (Fig. 14.5).

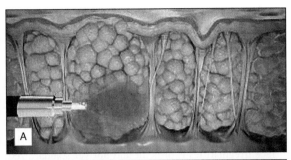

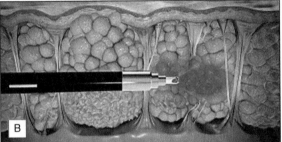

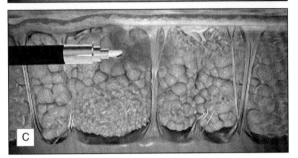

Figure 14.4 Schematic representation of the three-part Cellulaze™ treatment process: **(A)** denaturation of hypodermal adipocytes, **(B)** denaturation of dermal septa, and **(C)** stimulation of hypodermal tissue *(with permission of Cynosure Inc., Chelmsford, MA)*

More recently published studies by DiBernardo et al.[23] and Katz[24] were able to confirm these first results. The studies further showed that in 90–95% of the cases blinded evaluators were able to distinguish baseline photographs from those taken after the treatment. At 6 months post-treatment, blinded evaluators rated at least a 1-point improvement in the appearance of cellulite in 94–96% of treated sites. Katz[24] further showed that the average decrease in dimple depth based on absolute dimple depth values was 42% at 3 months and 49% at 6 months. Overall both patients and physicians reported satisfaction with the clinical outcome.

> **Pearl 3**
>
> Minimally invasive laser treatments appear to be most effective and may yield a permanent improvement.

Long-pulsed 1064 nm Nd:YAG laser

The long-pulsed 1064 nm Nd:YAG laser has been used to treat the appearance of cellulite, as an off-label use. This wavelength achieves a penetration depth of up to 4 cm, and has been extensively reported to efficiently induce neocollagenesis. Presumably, neocollagenesis at the subcuticular junction may decrease the herniation of fat globules into the dermis, which is the basis for cellulite.

In a proof-of-concept protocol, 22 female subjects with cellulite of the lower extremities were treated with the long-pulsed Nd:YAG laser.[25] Subjects were randomized to receive higher energy treatment with cryogen spray cooling (CSC) (10 mm spot size; 50 J/cm²; 50 ms pulse duration and CSC settings of 30 ms duration with a 20 ms delay) or lower energy treatment with no CSC (10 mm; 20 J/cm²; 50 ms). Subjects received three

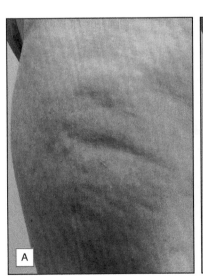

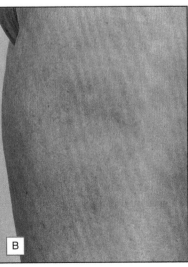

Figure 14.5 The left lateral thigh treated with the Cellulaze™ at **(A)** baseline, and **(B)** 6 months after treatment *(with permission of B. DiBernado, MD)*

treatments at 4-week intervals. Digital photographs and circumference measurements were taken pre-treatment and up to 6 months post-treatment. While no statistically significant difference was demonstrated for thigh circumference, blinded evaluators noted mild improvement in three of seven subjects in high energy group and moderate improvement in two of nine subjects in low energy group.[25]

Pearl 4

Maintenance treatments may be helpful for continued improvement.

Combination therapy

The application of a combination topical and light-based approach in the treatment of cellulite has also been attempted. In one pilot, split-design, randomized study, subjects with lower extremity cellulite applied phosphatidylcholine topical gel combined with LED of red (660 nm) and near-infrared (950 nm) wavelengths to one thigh, with placebo and LED to the contralateral thigh.[26] Greater improvement was observed in the combination phosphatidylcholine/LED-treated thighs as compared with the placebo/LED-treated thighs.[26]

Future research

Potential future areas of research employing laser and light-based technology include the application of near-infrared wavelengths to induce neocollagenesis at the subcuticular junction. The author (MAA) is in the process of employing an infrared broadband device (800–1600 nm; NIR, Alma Lasers) for the treatment of cellulite of the thighs and buttocks (unpublished results). Two additional areas of future research include facilitated delivery methods and photodynamic therapy as methods of boosting therapeutic efficacy. In the case of facilitated delivery, a fractional resurfacing device may be used to deliver a compound that boosts efficacy with subsequent laser and light-based technologies. Alternatively, a lipophilic photosensitizer may be combined with a laser or light of a deeply penetrating wavelength to boost adipocyte programmed cell death. Further exploration of combination therapies to enhance efficacy using facilitated delivery, topical application of a fat metabolizer or photosensitizer concomitant with laser or light-based therapy will provide future avenues of exploration in the treatment of cellulite.

Conclusion

In summary, the use of light-based devices in the treatment of cellulite is rapidly increasing in aesthetic dermatology. The devices that are currently available in the US include devices emitting green (532 nm), red (650 nm) and infrared (700–2000 nm) laser and/or broadband light, that are used at a low- or high-energy level. Several devices incorporate concomitant mechanical manipulation of the tissue.

Although numerous studies are available evaluating light-based treatment modalities to improve the appearance of cellulite, the level of proven efficacy remains unsatisfactory in the published literature. Limitations include relatively small sample sizes as well as the absence of control groups and comparative studies in general. Moreover, since photographic documentation of skin surface irregularities is difficult and not yet standardized, the lack of quantifiable, objective assessment methods is still a key problem. Additionally, while short-term clinical effects are encouraging, long-term results have not yet been proven with any of the medical devices available. Therefore, substantial research and further development is needed in order to confirm long-term effectiveness.

CASE STUDY 1

The patient is a 39-year-old white female who presents with cellulite on her thighs. She first noticed the condition in her early 30s, but it has worsened over time. An avid biker, she reports being unable to improve the condition through exercise. The patient is unwilling to pursue invasive treatments, and instead is interested in noninvasive options to improve the appearance of her thigh cellulite.

Physical examination reveals highly toned musculature of the lower extremities. The overlying skin is significant for diffuse, moderate dimpling in the gluteal-femoral regions.

Education is provided regarding the various treatment options, including no treatment, plastic surgery options, liposuction, laser-assisted liposuction, and laser and light-based treatments. Given the lack of substantive fat, the patient is not a good candidate for liposuction or laser-assisted liposuction. Following consultation and discussion of the treatment options, the patient opts for a noninvasive approach. A total of 14 biweekly treatments with an 808 nm diode low-level laser (TriActive, Cynosure Inc., Chelmsford) are administered. Each treatment was painless with minimal erythema and no adverse events.

The patient achieves modest improvement as assessed by the physician using the Visual Cellulite Grading Scale. This patient tolerated her treatments well with no complications.

CASE STUDY 2

A 50-year-old white female patient presents complaining of long-standing cellulite of the thighs. The patient exercises regularly. However, the condition has worsened in her postmenopausal years. She is unwilling to undergo invasive treatments and is only interested in noninvasive options to improve the appearance of her thighs.

Physical examination is significant for extensive dimpling and a 'cottage cheese' appearance to the bilateral thighs, most pronounced in the gluteal-femoral regions.

CASE STUDY 2—Continued

Education is provided regarding the various treatment options for cellulite, including no treatment, plastic surgery options, liposuction, and laser and light-based treatments. Given that the patient has ruled out invasive forms of treatment, laser and light-based options are discussed further and the patient opts to pursue a noninvasive treatment strategy.

Treatment is administered with a combination red light, radiofrequency and vacuum massage device (VelaShape III, Syneron). A total of 5 biweekly treatments are performed on the bilateral thighs. Each treatment was painless with minimal erythema and no adverse events.

The patient achieves modest improvement in the degree of dimpling of her cellulite in the gluteal-femoral regions of her lower extremities. In addition, the physician measures a 1 cm reduction in thigh circumference per thigh. Treatment was tolerated well with no complications (see Fig. 14.2).

References

1. Nürnberger F, Müller G. So-called cellulite: an invented disease. J Dermatol Surg Oncol 1978;4:221–9.

2. Piérard GE, Nizet JL, Piérard-Franchimont C. Cellulite: from standing fat herniation to hypodermal stretch marks. Am J Dermatopathol 2000;22:34–7.

3. Emanuele E. Cellulite: advances in treatment: facts and controversies. Clin Dermatol 2013;31:725–30.

4. Hexsel DM, Abreu M, Rodrigues TC, et al. Side-by-side comparison of areas with and without cellulite depressions using magnetic resonance imaging. Dermatol Surg 2009;35:1471–7.

5. Neira R, Arroyave J, Ramirez H, et al. Fat liquefaction: effect of low-level laser energy on adipose tissue. Plast Reconstr Surg 2002;110:912–25.

6. Nestor MS, Newburger J, Zarraga MB. Body contouring using 635-nm low level laser therapy. Semin Cutan Med Surg 2013;32:35–40.

7. Sadick NS, Mulholland RS. A prospective clinical study to evaluate the efficacy and safety of cellulite treatment using the combination of optical and RF energies for subcutaneous tissue heating. J Cosmet Laser Ther 2004;6:187–90.

8. Gold MH. Cellulite – an overview of non-invasive therapy with energy-based systems. J Dtsch Dermatol Ges 2012;10:553–8.

9. Sadick NS. Overview of ultrasound-assisted liposuction, and body contouring with cellulite reduction. Semin Cutan Med Surg 2009;28:250–6.

10. Wanitphakdeedecha R, Manuskiatti W. Treatment of cellulite with a bipolar radiofrequency, infrared heat, and pulsatile suction device: a pilot study. J Cosmet Dermatol 2006;5: 284–8.

11. Alster TS, Tanzi EL. Cellulite treatment using a novel combination radiofrequency, infrared light, and mechanical tissue manipulation device. J Cosmet Laser Ther 2005;7:81–5.

12. Romero C, Caballero N, Herrero M, et al. Effects of cellulite treatment with RF, IR light, mechanical massage and suction treating one buttock with the contralateral as a control. J Cosmet Laser Ther 2008;10:193–201.

13. Gold M. The use of rhythmic suction massage, low level laser irradiation, and superficial cooling to effect changes in adipose tissue/cellulite. Lasers Surg Med 2006;38(Suppl.):65.

14. Boyce S, Pabby A, Brazzini B, et al. Clinical evaluation of a device for the treatment of cellulite: TriActive. Am J Cosmet Surg 2005;22:233–7.

15. Nootheti PK, Magpantay A, Yosowitz G, et al. A single center, randomized, comparative, prospective clinical study to determine the efficacy of the VelaSmooth™ system versus the TriActive system for the treatment of cellulite. Lasers Surg Med 2006;38:908–12.

16. Jackson RF, Roche GC, Shanks SC. A double-blind, placebo-controlled randomized trial evaluating the ability of low-level laser therapy to improve the appearance of cellulite. Lasers Surg Med 2013;45:141–7.

17. Anderson RR, Farinelli W, Laubach H, et al. Selective photothermolysis of lipid-rich tissues: a free electron laser study. Lasers Surg Med 2006;38:913–19.

18. Collis N, Elliot LA, Sharpe C, Sharpe DT. Cellulite treatment: a myth or reality: a prospective randomized, controlled trial of two therapies, endermologie and aminophylline cream. Plast Reconstr Surg 1999;104:1110–17.

19. Gold MH, Khatri KA, Hails K, et al. Reduction in thigh circumference and improvement in the appearance of cellulite with dual-wavelength, low-level laser energy and massage. J Cosmet Laser Ther 2011;13:13–20.

20. Lach E. Reduction of subcutaneous fat and improvement in cellulite appearance by dual-wavelength, low-level laser energy combined with vacuum and massage. J Cosmet Laser Ther 2008;10:202–9.

21. Kulick MI. Evaluation of a noninvasive, dual-wavelength laser-suction and massage device for the regional treatment of cellulite. Plast Reconstr Surg 2010;25:1788–96.

22. DiBernardo BE. Treatment of cellulite using a 1440-nm pulsed laser with one-year follow-up. J Am Soc Aesthetic Plast Surg 2011;31:328–41.

23. DiBernardo B, Sasaki G, Katz BE, et al. A multicenter study for a single, three-step laser treatment for cellulite using a 1440-nm Nd:YAG laser, a novel side-firing fiber, and a temperature-sensing cannula. J Am Soc Aesthetic Plast Surg 2013;33:576–84.

24. Katz B. Quantitative and qualitative evaluation of the efficacy of a 1440 nm Nd:YAG laser with novel bi-directional optical fiber in the treatment of cellulite as measured by 3-dimensional surface imaging. J Drugs Dermatol 2013;12:1224–30.

25. Truitt A, Elkeeb L, Ortiz A, et al. Evaluation of a long pulsed 1064-nm Nd:YAG laser for improvement in appearance of cellulite. J Cosmet Laser Ther 2012;14:139–44.

26. Sasaki GH, Oberg K, Tucker B, Gaston M. The effectiveness and safety of topical PhotoActif phosphatidylcholine-based anti-cellulite gel and LED (red and near-infrared) light on grade II-III thigh cellulite: a randomized, double-blinded study. J Cosmet Laser Ther 2007;9:87–96.

Radiofrequency and Ultrasound: Cellulite Reduction

15

Emily C. Keller, Arielle N.B. Kauvar

Key Messages

- Radiofrequency and ultrasound devices are at the forefront of medical advances in the treatment of cellulite
- Radiofrequency generates heat in the tissue, resulting in shrinkage of collagen fibers, stimulation of new collagen and elastin, and destruction of adipocytes
- Ultrasound uses focused sound waves to cause mechanical and thermal damage to the tissue, resulting in lysis of adipocytes, stimulation of collagen and improvement in circulation
- Although these devices may provide improvement in the appearance of cellulite, the results are temporary; no lasting improvements have been achieved
- Patients who receive the most benefit from these devices often have a moderate amount of cellulite on the buttocks or the thighs, have little skin laxity, maintain a healthy weight, and are capable of returning for a series of treatments

Cellulite

Cellulite is the lay term used to describe puckered or dimpled skin, most often present on the thighs and buttocks of women, and has been termed liposclerosis, gynoid dystrophy, dermopanniculitis, and edematofibrosclerosis in the medical literature.[1] Cellulite is considered a normal physiologic state of secondary sex characteristics in females, 85–98% of whom are affected, regardless of their BMI.

Histologic studies demonstrate that the appearance of cellulite relates to the architecture of the skin and subcutis in affected skin. Fibrous septa in women extend from the dermis to deep fascia in a perpendicular pattern, resembling a mattress or down quilt, in contrast with those of men, where they form a criss-cross pattern. As the fat layer expands, pockets of fat herniate into the reticular and papillary dermis and are fixed in place by the fibrous septa. As the skin thins with age, the herniated fat becomes more evident.[2] The pathophysiology of cellulite is multifactorial and complex. Cellulite is stimulated by estrogens. There is also evidence that cellulite may worsen when the microcirculation and lymphatic drainage are compromised.[1] A more extensive discussion of the pathophysiology of cellulite can be found in Chapter 12.

Treatments aimed at fat reduction such as liposuction, high intensity focused ultrasound, and cryolipolysis, cannot target fat herniations associated with cellulite because of the risk of necrosis of the thin overlying skin. Many of the invasive and noninvasive therapies developed for cellulite treatment use a combination of modalities designed to correct the architectural and physiologic abnormalities that are thought to contribute to cellulite formation (Box 15.1). These include lysing or evacuating the superficial adipocytes, increasing the metabolic activity of the adipocytes via heat or norepinephrine secretion, decreasing lymphedema, increasing the thickness of the skin by inducing new collagen formation and remodeling, and altering the fibrous septa.[3]

Many of the technologies that will be discussed below lack controlled trials, and those that have been studied often were examined in investigations that have clinical endpoints that are difficult to reproduce, such as circumferential reduction and inconsistent photography. Objective evidence of improvement such as MRI studies is uncommon, and cellulite improvement is often difficult to assess, even with standardized photography.

Box 15.1
Proposed mechanism of action in cellulite treatments

Increased blood circulation
Realignment of collagen fibrils
Thickening of collagen fibers
Thickening and shortening of fibrous septa
Dermal fibrosis
Neocollagenesis
Release of messenger enzymes from adipocytes
Lipolysis

Radiofrequency

Radiofrequ;ency (RF) has been used in medicine for many years to electrodesiccate, coagulate, and ablate tissue. RF relies on heating of water rather than absorption by tissue chromophores, and hence can be used in any skin type. RF creates an oscillating electrical current which induces collisions between charged ions and molecules in tissue, resulting in the generation of heat. The biologic effects of the tissue heating vary depending on the frequency used, depth of delivery, and selectivity achieved with skin cooling. The depth of penetration of RF is inversely proportional to the frequency, and the relative degree of heating of water or fat will depend on the electric field.

RF treatment of skin produces temporary shrinkage of collagen molecules, and stimulation of new collagen and elastin production. The amount of tissue contraction and remodeling is dependent upon the maximum temperature reached, the length of time that temperature is maintained, and the conductivity and age of the tissue.[4] Collagen remodels and neocollagenesis is induced when the reticular dermis reaches 60–65 °C, which correlates with a surface temperature of 40–42 °C, the target temperature of RF devices.[5] RF can also be used to heat and destroy fat. Heating of adipocytes with RF increases adipocyte apoptosis as well as lipase-mediated enzymatic degradation of triglycerides into free fatty acids and glycerol.[3]

RF may be delivered using monopolar, bipolar, or unipolar devices, alone or in combination with other technologies. With monopolar devices, patients are grounded and the RF is delivered via the skin to the grounding electrode. RF travels best through tissues with high water content and produces the greatest resistance in fat, creating the highest temperature rise. Monopolar RF is delivered in a stamped mode with individual pulses or in a continuous mode, where the handpiece is applied to the skin with constant motion.

Bipolar RF is less deeply penetrating than monopolar RF. The RF travels between two poles (positive to negative), and the distance between the electrodes determines the depth of penetration in tissue, which is typically 1–4 mm. With unipolar RF, there is a single electrode without a grounding pad. The RF is emitted in all directions around the electrode. Unipolar RF uses high-frequency electromagnetic radiation at 40 MHz, not electrical current, to cause oscillation of water molecules to produce heat. The penetration ranges from 15 to 20 mm.[6,7] Tripolar RF is a variation that uses a combination monopolar and bipolar electrode.[4]

Pearl 1

A surface temperature of 40–42 °C must be achieved in order for RF energy to cause an alteration in collagen fibers.

Ultrasound

Ultrasound is a mechanical compression or sound wave that is above the audible range (>20 kHz) and may destroy fat cells by mechanical or thermal mechanisms.[8] Ultrasound is characterized by its frequency in kiloHertz (kHz) or megaHertz (MHz) and intensity in W/cm^2. Like other electromagnetic radiation, ultrasound travels through tissue and is reflected, absorbed, or scattered. Waves are propagated through tissue causing molecules to oscillate and create energy that is transformed into heat.[9] These repeated movements cause cavitation, which results in mechanical disruption and eventual death of the target cells.[8,9]

In tissue, ultrasound becomes increasingly attenuated with higher frequencies, resulting in less depth of penetration. Ultrasound is commonly employed for diagnostic purposes, using frequencies in the range of 2–20 MHz. This type of ultrasound, termed 'nonfocused', delivers low-energy, diffuse waves that do not produce a sufficient amount of heat in the tissue to cause destruction. For body contouring, fat removal and improvement in cellulite, ultrasound is 'focused', with frequencies in the range of 0.8–3.5 MHz. The focused nature of waves allows for energy to be directed at a small region or single point, resulting in heat or mechanical disruption to cause tissue damage. Thus, the subcutaneous fat may be treated, while the critical surrounding structures are left unharmed.[10]

When directing treatment to improving the appearance of cellulite, devices often use a medium-intensity ultrasound. This allows for propagation of the signal to reach the subcutaneous fat, but also provides some spread of energy to the surrounding collagen. Ultrasound energy causes lysis of fat cells, but also stimulates collagen thickening by heating the dermis and improves circulation. Studies have also shown that ultrasound results in breakdown of fat secondary to secretion of norepinephrine from sympathetic nerves.[11]

Patient selection

The prototypical patient has moderate cellulite on the buttocks and thighs. Ideally, the contour abnormalities could be captured with standardized photography.[12] Patients should be prepared to return for a series of treatments within a reasonable timeframe. Their expectations should be managed and they should be educated about the likelihood of delayed improvement.

Contraindications for RF devices include implanted electronic and metal devices, pregnancy, current use of isotretinoin, hip surgery or replacement, treatment over tattoos or permanent makeup/filler, blood dyscrasia or diseases with altered collagen-vascular properties.[4]

Contraindications for ultrasound-based devices include pregnancy (exclusion of any region near the fetus); thrombophlebitis or thromboembolic disease; treatment over the vertebrae; treatment in the thoracic region if a pacemaker is present; treatment around the eye; treatment over bony fractures, metal implants, hip surgery or replacement; and current malignancy (to avoid tissue disruption and unwanted increased spread of malignant cells). Caution should be used when treating over bony prominences or regions with decreased sensitivity.

Side effects

Although infrequent, burns and fat atrophy may occur. Patients need to be properly grounded at all times and the cooling devices must be functioning properly. Fat atrophy is often a result of using energies that are too high or repeatedly treating an area without allowing for cooling. Overall, the safety profiles of these devices are excellent, and, if used properly, they are associated with few side effects or complications.

Pearl 2

The use of standardized photography is essential in determining the efficacy of these treatments.

Radiofrequency devices

Monopolar radiofrequency devices

Thermage®

Thermage® (Solta Medical Inc., Hayward, CA) is a monopolar RF device FDA-approved for the noninvasive treatment of rhytides and the temporary improvement in the appearance of cellulite (Table 15.1). The device has a

Table 15.1 Devices used to treat cellulite

Device	Modality
Thermage®	Monopolar RF
VelaSmooth™	Bipolar RF
VelaShape™	Bipolar RF
Reaction™	Bipolar RF
Accent™ RF System	Unipolar or bipolar RF
TriPollar™	Tripolar RF
Venus Freeze™	Multipolar RF
C-Actor®	Ultrasound
VASERshape™	Ultrasound
Bella Contour®	Ultrasound
UltraShape	Ultrasound
Ulthera	Ultrasound

generator, a handpiece with treatment tip, and a cryogen unit. The handpiece is equipped with sensors for skin temperature and pressure, as well as a cooling apparatus. Tip sizes vary depending on the treatment region, with the DC and CL tips used for body contouring and cellulite. The company supplies a temporary grid that may be applied to the patient's skin in order to provide a systematic treatment approach. Contact gel is spread over the area and, as the handpiece is activated, the epidermis is heated to 40–42 °C. Multiple passes are conducted over the treatment area, though care needs to be taken to allow epidermal cooling between passes.

Mechanism of action

The heat produced by monopolar RF (6 MHz) causes heat damage to collagen and incites the inflammatory cascade that results in a wound healing response. As RF produces volumetric heating, the collagen fibrils quickly shorten, providing the immediate appearance of tightening. The shrinkage is secondary to a breakdown of hydrogen bonds in the collagen chain. Blood flow is also increased which in turn allows for enhanced metabolism of fat. Over weeks to months, neocollagenesis occurs as a result of the wound healing response.[13,14]

Results

The majority of Thermage studies have been conducted to provide data for improvement of rhytides and facial laxity, with very few concentrating on body contouring and cellulite. Anolik et al.[15] conducted a blinded, multicenter trial using the ThermaCool TC to treat mild to moderate abdominal skin laxity in 12 patients. The protocol used the Thermage Multiplex Tip and most patients received 300 pulses with energies ranging from 28 to 46 J/cm^2. Of the patients who returned for follow-up, all had a decrease in waist circumference (body contour and skin laxity). All but one patient had aesthetic improvement (body contour and skin laxity). Patients received anxiolytics and analgesics before the procedure and side effects included transient edema and erythema, lasting only a few hours.[15]

Zelickson et al.[16] evaluated histologic specimens after Thermage treatment that revealed an increased diameter of collagen fibrils post-treatment. Protein analysis confirmed neocollagenesis by the presence of increased collagen type I mRNA expression.[16]

Side effects using the original system included fat atrophy, erosions, and dysesthesias. As new software and protocols were implemented that use lower-energy, higher-pass treatments, side effects have diminished significantly and patients typically experience only mild erythema and edema.

Exilis

Exilis (BTL Industries, Boston, MA) is an FDA-approved device for treatment of wrinkles and rhytides and is often used off-label for body shaping and skin tightening. The system incorporates monopolar RF with energy flow control (EFC). EFC is an innovative technology that eliminates energy peaks, allowing for a more controlled and constant heating of the tissue. BTL has coined this process as square ('flat top') spectrum energy profiling. As the handpiece allows for real-time monitoring of skin temperature and RF energy, the system will shut off if skin temperatures and energies are out of range. Patients usually receive four treatments, 1 week apart. There are no published clinical trials using this device for the treatment of cellulite, but there are anecdotal reports of improvement.[17]

Bipolar radiofrequency devices

VelaSmooth™

VelaSmooth™ (Syneron Medical Ltd, Yokneam, Israel) is an FDA-approved device that uses electrical optical synergy (ELOS) technology for noninvasive body contouring and improvement of cellulite. It combines infrared (IR) light (700–2000 nm), bipolar RF (up to 35 W) and massage with suction (750 mmHg negative pressure).

Mechanism of action

The heating of fat with a combination of two modalities is thought to increase fat metabolism by dissociating oxygen from oxyhemoglobin. The IR light preheats the tissue, to which RF is drawn, and since the RF is more easily conducted through heated tissue, less energy is required.[6] The IR penetrates to a depth of up to 3 mm and the RF portion reaches 2–20 mm.[18,19] The suction and massage rollers rupture fat cell clusters and manipulate the vertical fibrous septa, both of which contribute to the improved skin appearance of cellulite.[18] The device is used with a conductive lotion that is manufactured by the company.

Results

VelaSmooth has been shown to improve the appearance of cellulite in several studies. After a single treatment, histologic studies show that the VelaSmooth causes membrane rupture and incipient necrosis of adipocytes.[20]

In a split body study, Romero et al.[21] treated 10 patients with cellulite on the buttocks for a total of 12 sessions performed biweekly. The handpiece had an adjustable intensity, from 0–3, and all of the patients were treated at the highest intensity. Sessions lasted approximately 30 minutes and included 6–8 passes on one buttock. All patients had improvement in the appearance of cellulite, though results had decreased at the 2-month follow-up period. Following treatment, histologic analysis showed a realignment of the collagen fibers parallel to the dermal–epidermal junction and tightening of the dermal collagen, both of which contributed to the appearance of smoother skin texture.

VelaSmooth was studied by Kulick in 16 patients with cellulite on the posterior or lateral thigh, receiving biweekly treatments for 4 weeks.[22] Patients reported a

75% improvement in cellulite appearance at 3 months and 50% at 6 months. The investigators noted 62% improvement at 3 months and 50% at 6 months. The improvement achieved from the treatments appeared to be relatively short-lived and monthly maintenance treatments were required to sustain the improvement.

As both of the above studies noted a decreased degree of improvement as time since treatment increased, it is thought that monthly treatments may be necessary for maintenance.

Pearl 3

Providers may want to emphasize to patients that results are temporary and patients may need to have additional treatments over time to maintain results.

VelaShape™

VelaShape™, the second generation of the VelaSmooth, is FDA-approved for circumferential reduction and for the treatment of cellulite (Fig. 15.1). It incorporates ELOS technology with massage and suction, but provides higher treatment energies resulting in treatment durations that are approximately 30% shorter as compared to the VelaSmooth.[18]

Mechanism of action

The mechanism of action is identical to that of the VelaSmooth, though the IR and RF energies available for treatment are higher. The VelaShape comes with two handpieces: the VelaSmooth handpiece for larger areas and the VelaContour® handpiece for smaller treatment areas.[23] The VelaContour handpiece provides peak IR energy at 20 W and RF energy at 23 W.[23] The VelaShape II has 20% more power than the original device (RF 60 W) and VelaShape III has a maximum RF of 150 W, which enables decreased treatment duration and number of sessions.

Results

Brightman et al.[24] noted improvement in cellulite appearance in arms and post-partum abdominal and flank regions with the VelaShape in a nonrandomized clinical trial. Arms were treated weekly for five sessions and the abdomen and flank were treated during four weekly sessions. Energy settings were RF at 50 W, IR at 20 W and suction at 750 mmHg negative pressure. Skin temperature was maintained at 40–42 °C for 5 minutes to achieve the highest chance for collagen denaturation. Histology confirmed an increase in both fibroblasts and collagen fibers. Patients experienced ecchymoses that resolved within 60 minutes post-treatment.

Winter conducted a prospective, self-controlled study using the VelaShape in 20 women with cellulite on the abdomen, buttocks and thighs.[19] The women received five

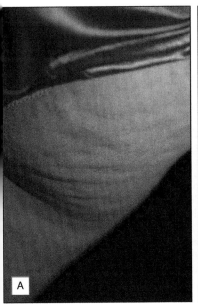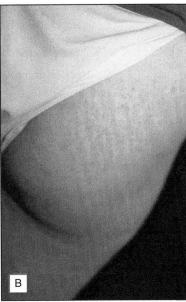

A

B

Figure 15.1 Improvement in the appearance of cellulite after eight treatment sessions with the VelaShape *(courtesy of J. Shaoul, MD)*

weekly treatments and all had statistically significant improvement in cellulite.

The VelaShape device was used in a histologic analysis study by Hexsel and colleagues in nine patients with cellulite on the posterior thighs and buttocks.[25] Patients were required to complete a total of 12 sessions via six biweekly treatments that lasted 60 minutes. There was statistically significant improvement in cellulite of the buttocks, but not on the thighs, though some positive change was noted even there.

Reaction™

Reaction™ (Viora Inc., Jersey City, NJ) uses bipolar RF and massage with channeling optimized radiofrequency energy (CORE) technology. Three RF frequencies (0.8 MHz, 1.7 MHz, 2.45 MHz) and four vacuum levels allow the user to customize the depth of penetration. The device is FDA-approved for cellulite treatment and comes with three different applicators for varying treatment fields and locations.

Mechanism of action

The Reaction device produces improvement in the appearance of cellulite via tissue heating, achieving epidermal skin temperatures of 40–42 °C. Heat induces shrinkage of fat cells and increases blood circulation to stimulate fibroblasts and production of new collagen.

Results

Twenty-four patients with cellulite on the abdomen, thighs, and buttocks were treated with eight weekly sessions, each session lasting 20 minutes. Tissue temperature ranged from 39 °C to 42 °C. Evaluation confirmed increased blood flow and new formation of connective tissue. Overall, patients had a 55% improvement in cellulite appearance, which was sustained for 3 months.[4]

Combination unipolar and bipolar radiofrequency devices

Accent™ RF system

Accent™ RF system (Alma Lasers Ltd, Buffalo Grove, IL) incorporates both unipolar and bipolar RF handpieces. It is used off-label for the treatment of cellulite. The unipolar handpiece penetrates up to 20 mm, whereas the bipolar handpiece penetrates 2–4 mm.[5]

Mechanism of action

Accent RF system is thought to improve the appearance of cellulite by causing dermal fibrosis. The unipolar handpiece produces volumetric heating and the multipolar handpiece provides controlled surface heating. The heat induces neocollagenesis and collagen remodeling. There may also be an increase in the amount of elastin production.

Results

Alexiades-Armenakas et al.[5] conducted a randomized, blinded, split-design study of the Accent unipolar handpiece in 10 patients with cellulite on the thighs. All patients received six treatments at 2-week intervals.[5] After mineral oil was applied, the handpiece was moved in a circular motion to achieve a skin temperature of 40–43 °C at an RF of 150–200 W. This was followed by three 30-second passes at decrements of 10 W. Patients experienced erythema that lasted 1–3 hours post-treatment. The greatest improvement was seen in dimple density (11.25% improvement) and the least was noted in dimple depth (1.75–2.5% improvement). The mean overall cellulite improvement was 8%, though this was not statistically significant.

The unipolar handpiece was also studied by del Pino in 26 females with cellulite on the buttocks and thighs who received two treatments 15 days apart.[26] The sessions consisted of three 30-second passes and ultrasound was used to evaluate the skin thickness. There was a distinct decrease in distance from the stratum corneum to Camper's fascia; 68% of patients had volume contraction of approximately 20%. The study confirmed that high-energy RF induced changes in the fibrous septa.

Goldberg and colleagues also evaluated the efficacy of the Accent RF system in a study of 30 patients with cellulite on the thighs.[7] Patients received a total of six treatments, delivered every other week. Sessions were 30 minutes in duration, delivering 150–170 W and reaching a skin temperature of 40–42 °C. Patients experienced erythema that lasted up to 2 hours. Ninety percent of patients had clinical improvement in the appearance of cellulite. The analysis suggests that the immediately observed improvement results from collagen contraction and longer term changes result from dermal fibrosis.

Pearl 4

The study conducted by del Pino[26] was pivotal in confirming that high-energy RF has the capacity to heat deep subcutaneous tissue and provide significant contraction of collagen.

Tripolar radiofrequency devices

TriPollar™

TriPollar™ (Pollogen, Tel Aviv, Israel) uses three electrodes to combine bipolar and monopolar RF (5–30 W) into one handpiece, reaching up to 20 mm depth, in order to produce immediate collagen contraction and stimulate new collagen formation.[23] There are two different treatment tips that may be interchanged for large or small treatment areas.[27] Cooling of the skin surface is not necessary during treatment with this device.

Mechanism of action

The TriPollar uses the combined energy of bipolar and monopolar RF to cause volumetric heating, which in turn produces immediate contraction of collagen and neocollagenesis. As the fibrous bands thicken, fat herniation is minimized and the appearance of the skin is smoother.

Results

Manuskiatti and colleagues conducted a pilot study that used the TriPollar device to treat 39 females with cellulite on the abdomen, thighs, buttocks, and arms during eight weekly sessions.[28] After applying glycerin oil, 20 W RF and 28.5 W RF were used to heat the skin to 40–42 °C for 2 minutes. Sessions lasted 30–60 minutes, depending on the treatment area. Patients had a 50% improvement in cellulite appearance. Side effects included mild erythema that lasted 2–3 hours post-treatment and mild prickling and heat during treatment.

Kaplan and Gat[27] treated 12 patients with an average of seven weekly treatments on the face, neck, arms, and abdomen to determine if the TriPollar would decrease fat and stimulate collagen. Histologic analysis confirmed an increase in dermal thickness as a result of collagen fiber thickening and shrinkage of fat cells.

Multipolar radiofrequency devices

Venus Freeze™

Venus Freeze™ (Venus Concepts, Karmiel, Israel) is a device that encompasses multipolar RF and pulsed magnetic fields to provide improvement in the appearance of cellulite. Venus Concepts has dubbed their technology (MP)²®: Multi Polar Magnetic Pulses[29] (Fig. 15.2). The device is FDA approved for facial wrinkles and rhytides in the US and licensed in Canada for temporary treatment of cellulite.[30]

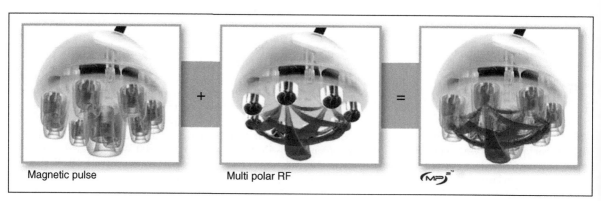

Magnetic pulse   +   Multi polar RF   =   (MP)²

Figure 15.2 Venus Freeze (MP)² technology: combination of pulsed magnetic fields and multipolar RF *(courtesy of Venus Concepts)*

BUTTOCKS AND THIGHS

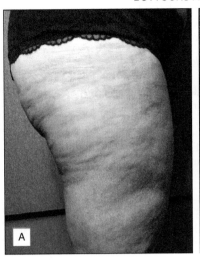

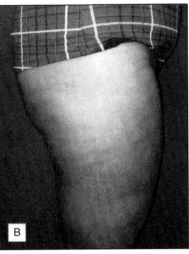

Figure 15.3 Improvement in the appearance of cellulite after eight treatment sessions with the Venus Freeze *(courtesy of Body Care by Angie, Canada)*

Mechanism of action

(MP)[2] technology produces deep heating to stimulate collagen remodeling, architectural changes in the adipose tissue and neovascularity to assist in remodeling and regeneration.[31] The device comes with two applicators, one with eight multipolar electrodes and the other with four multipolar electrodes that may be used on different sized treatment areas.[32]

Results

The company website provides two patient-assessed clinical trials and there is a current trial to evaluate the efficacy in cellulite treatment (Fig. 15.3).

Thirty-five patients were treated on the abdomen, buttocks, thighs and arms in order to achieve skin tightening and cellulite improvement.[30] They received once weekly treatments for 6–10 weeks; each treatment lasted 20–60 minutes. Patients noted improvement in cellulite after the first treatment and there were no significant side effects.

Another trial treated eight patients for cellulite.[32] After glycerin was applied to the skin, the applicators were moved constantly over the skin to reach a goal temperature of 40–42 °C, which was maintained for 10 minutes. Seventy-five percent of patients noted improvement in the appearance of cellulite.

Ultrasound devices

CELLACTOR® SC1

C-Actor® of the CELLACTOR® SC1 (Storz Medical AG, Tagerwilen, Switzerland) is a device that uses extracorporeal pulse activation therapy (EPAT) to treat cellulite. This is akin to acoustic wave therapy used in urology and orthopedics to treat kidney stones and joint calcifications.

Mechanism of action

EPAT stimulates microcirculation and improves cell permeability. Fat cells are able to release phospholipases, inducing lipolysis. The elastic and collagen fibers thicken, causing the dermis to become denser. Oxidative stress is diminished and antioxidants are increased.[33]

Results

In a randomized, controlled study, Christ et al.[33] treated 59 women with advanced cellulite on the thighs and gluteal region with three biweekly or four biweekly sessions. Ultrasound gel was applied to the treatment area and 800 pulses were delivered at an average of 0.25 mJ/mm[2] by moving the treatment tip horizontally and vertically. Those who received six treatments achieved a 75% increase in skin elasticity at the 3-month follow-up. Those who received eight treatments noted a 95% improvement 3 months post-procedure. Side effects included mild pain and redness during treatment sessions. Histology confirmed an increase in the density of collagen and elastic fibers, neocollagenesis, and increased lipolysis.

Adatto and colleagues conducted a randomized, controlled study that noted the CELLACTOR SC1 improved cellulite in all 14 women treated with eight sessions in 4 weeks on the saddle-bag region.[34] They found that as blood flow is increased, the breakdown of fat is stimulated, whereas low blood flow causes fat storage. The authors suggest that CELLACTOR SC1 improves cellulite by altering the dermal microvasculature.

> **Pearl 5**
>
> In addition to causing lysis of adipocytes and stimulation of new collagen, ultrasound may increase microcirculation in the treatment region, allowing for more efficacious removal of adipocytes and improved lymphatic drainage.

Bella Contour®

Bella Contour® is FDA-approved for the temporary reduction in the appearance of cellulite. The device incorporates low intensity, nonfocused continuous wave ultrasound with electric fields and massage.[35] The transducer produces ultrasound frequencies from 0.8 MHz to 3.4 MHz and the four electrodes may be adjusted for varying degrees of intensity. Depth of penetration ranges from 0.2 to 4.0 cm.

Mechanism of action

The combination of ultrasound and electrical fields produces a mechanical effect on the adipose tissue, causing it to release fat, resulting in circumferential reduction and improvement in the appearance of cellulite.

Results

Reports have not been published and are from the company website. Treatment sessions often last 40 minutes: 20 minutes directed toward cellulite and skin appearance improvement and another 20 minutes for deep fat treatment. Based upon standardized photographs from the company, there is recognizable improvement in cellulite. These reports state that patients did not have any untoward side effects.

Ultrashape®

Ultrashape® (Ultrashape Inc., Yokneam, Israel) is a nonthermal, focused ultrasound pulsed-wave device used for selective fat lipolysis. The device is not FDA-approved for cellulite, though patients have seen improvement in the appearance of cellulite.[3,36] The Ultrashape Contour I houses a transducer for focused US waves, temperature sensors, and an acoustic monitor.[10]

Mechanism of action

Ultrashape causes cavitation and eventual mechanical destruction of fat cells. The device uses mechanical energy, not thermal effects, to produce lysis of fat cells. The inflammatory cascade is stimulated to help clear damaged adipocytes.

Results

Histology confirms lipolysis of adipocytes with no harm to the surrounding tissues. The procedure consists of three treatments performed 2 weeks apart. Patients are encouraged to keep a negative caloric intake for 4 days post-treatment in order to metabolize the released fat.[8]

Ulthera

Ulthera® uses intense focused ultrasound (IFUS), operating at 4–7 MHz, to create small 1–1.5 mm thermal coagulation points (TCP) at precise depths. It is FDA cleared for skin tightening but has anecdotally been found to improve cellulite. The device consists of a central power unit and interchangeable handpieces. Each handpiece has a transducer that allows real time visualization of the dermis and subcutis, using unfocused low energy ultrasound, and treatment at high energy exposures that coagulates tissue. The individual handpieces focus at 1.5, 3.0 and 4.5 mm in depth. Each probe delivers the energy in a straight line, with adjustable power, exposure times and spacing of exposure zones.

Mechanism of action

There is histologic evidence of precise microcoagulation zones in the deep dermis and superficial musculoaponeurotic system. Treatment results in the generation of collagen and elastin, with resultant thickening of the reticular dermis and clinically apparent skin tightening. Ulthera received FDA clearance in 2009 for eyebrow lifting, and subsequent approval for neck and submental lifting.[37,38]

Results

The device is used off-label for the treatment of other body areas. A study by Alster and Tanzi demonstrated that treatment of arms, medial thighs and extensor knees resulted in statistically significant improvement in skin texture and contour 3–6 months following treatment. In each subject, one side was randomized to receive treatment with a 4 MHz, 4.5 mm focal depth transducer, and the other side was treated with both the 4 MHz, 4.5 mm focal depth transducer and the 7 MHz, 3.0 mm focal depth transducer. The dual plane treatment yielded slightly better scores. Side effects were limited to focal erythema, tenderness, and bruising lasting up to 1 week.[39]

The endpoint of this study was tissue 'tightening', but the observed improvement in contour and texture could conceivably improve the appearance of cellulite by means of dermal thickening. Treatment of cellulite is currently practically limited by the time required to treat larger skin areas.

VASERshape™

VASERshape™ (Sound Surgical Technologies LLC) is FDA approved for the temporary reduction in the appearance of cellulite.[40] The device contains two beams of overlapping ultrasound energy at 1 MHz and vacuum massage, allowing for 1–5 cm depth of penetration. Patients are encouraged to obtain 3–5 treatments once weekly, with 45–60 minutes allocated per treatment area (8.5 × 11 mm size). There are no peer-reviewed published reports available.

Conclusions

There are a wide variety of devices that have been developed for the treatment of cellulite. For many of these devices, controlled clinical trials are lacking. For those devices that have shown objective evidence of cellulite improvement, the results are often short-lived, and regular maintenance treatments are required. That being said, cellulite is a significant cosmetic concern for many women, so that even a temporary improvement is often desirable.

CASE STUDY 1

A 35-year-old female, JD, presents for cellulite of her outer thighs. She states that she has had visible cellulite of her thighs since her early twenties, as does her sister and mother. She participates in Pilates three times weekly, runs twice weekly, and maintains a healthy diet and weight. No matter how much exercising or dieting she does, she cannot get rid of her cellulite. She is interested in noninvasive means to improve her cellulite.

On physical examination, she has five discrete dells of the right and left outer thigh, as well as diffuse rippling of the outer thighs.

JD discusses treatment options with her provider, including laser/light-based devices, laser/liposuction, radiofrequency devices and ultrasound devices. Based on the topography of the cellulite and the patient's desire to avoid invasive treatments, the provider and patient agree on using the VelaShape II. Standardized photographs are obtained prior to treatment.

The patient undergoes five weekly treatments with the VelaShape II. Based on visual inspection and comparison with her pre-treatment photographs, JD acknowledges moderate improvement in the appearance of her cellulite. She reports having experienced erythema of the treatment areas that would last approximately 30 minutes post-treatment, but no other side effects.

References

1. Khan MH, Victor F, Rao B, Sadick NS. Treatment of cellulite. Part I: pathophysiology. JAAD 2010;62(3):361–70.
2. Nurnberger F, Muller G. So-called cellulite: an invented disease. J Dermatol Surg Oncol 1978;4(3):221–9.
3. Khan M, Victor F, Rao B, Sadick NS. Treatment of cellulite. Part II: advances and controveries. JAAD 2010;62(3):373–84.
4. Belenky I, Margulis A, Elman M, et al. Exploring optimized radiofrequency energy: a review of radiofrequency history and applications in esthetic fields. Adv Ther 2012; 29(3):249–66.
5. Alexiades-Armenakas M, Dover JS, Arndt KA. Unipolar radiofrequency treatment to improve the appearance of cellulite. J Cosmet Laser Ther 2008;10:148–53.
6. Lolis MS, Goldgerg DJ. Radiofrequency in cosmetic dermatology: a review. Dermatol Surg 2012;38:1765–76.
7. Goldberg DJ, Fazeli A, Berlin AL. Clinical, laboratory, and MRI analysis of cellulite treatment with a unipolar radiofrequency device. Dermatol Surg 2008;34(2):204–9.
8. Coleman KM, Coleman WP III, Benchetrit A. Non-invasive, external ultrasound lipolysis. Semin Cutan Med Surg 2009; 28:263–7.
9. Jewell ML, Solish NJ, Desilets CS. Noninvasive body sculpting technologies with an emphasis on high-intensity focused ultrasound. Aesth Plast Surg 2011;35:901–12.
10. Brown SA, Greenbaum L, Shtukmaster S, et al. Characterization of nonthermal focused ultrasound for noninvasive selective fat cell disruption (lysis): technical and preclinical assessment. Plast Reconstr Surg 2009;124(1): 92–101.
11. Miwa H, Kino M, Han LK, et al. Effect of ultrasound application on fat mobilization. Pathophysiology 2002;9:13–19.
12. Alster T, Tehrani M. Treatment of cellulite with optical devices: an overview with practical considerations. Lasers Surg Med 2006;38:727–30.
13. Sukal SA, Geronemus RG. Thermage: the nonablative radiofrequency for rejuvenation. Clin Dermatol 2008;26:602–7.
14. Hodgkinson DJ. Clinical applications of radiofrequency: nonsurgical skin tightening (thermage). Clin Plastic Surg 2009;36:261–8.
15. Anolik R, Chapas AM, Brightman LA, Geronemus RG. Radiofrequency devices for body shaping: a review and study of 12 patients. Semin Cutan Med Surg 2009;28:236–43.
16. Zelickson B, Kist D, Bernstein E, et al. Histological and ultrastructural evaluation of the effects of a radiofrequency-based non-ablative dermal remodeling device, a pilot study. Arch Dermatol 2004;140:204–9.
17. McDaniel D, Fritz K, Machovcova A, Bernardy J. A focused monopolar radiofrequency causes apoptosis: a porcine model. J Drugs Dermatol 2014;13(11):1336–40.
18. Sadick NS. Overview of ultrasound-assisted liposuction, and body contouring with cellulite reduction. Semin Cutan Med Surg 2009;28:250–6.
19. Winter ML. Post-pregnancy body contouring using a combined radiofrequency, infrared light and tissue manipulation device. J Cosmet Laser Ther 2009;11:229–35.
20. Trelles M, Mordon SR. Adipocyte membrane lysis observed after cellulite treatment is performed with radiofrequency. Aesth Plast Surg 2009;33:125–8.
21. Romero C, Caballero N, Herrero M, et al. Effects of cellulite treatment with RF, IR light, mechanical massage and suction treating one buttock with the contralateral as a control. J Cosmet Laser Ther 2008;10:193–201.
22. Kulick M. Evaluation of the combination of radio frequency, infrared energy and mechanical rollers with suction to improve skin surface irregularities (cellulite) in a limited treatment area. J Cosmet Laser Ther 2006;8:185–90.
23. Peterson JD, Goldman MP. Laser, light, and energy devices for cellulite and lipodystrophy. Clin Plastic Surg 2001;38:463–74.
24. Brightman L, Weiss E, Chapas AM, et al. Improvement in arm and post-partum abdominal and flank subcutaneous fat deposits and skin laxity using a bipolar radiofrequency, infrared, vacuum and mechanical massage device. Lasers Surg Med 2009;41:791–8.
25. Hexsel DM, Siega C, Schilling-Souza J, et al. A bipolar radiofrequency, infrared, vacuum and mechanical massage device for treatment of cellulite: a pilot study. J Cosmet Laser Ther 2011;13:297–302.
26. del Pino E, Rosado RH, Azuela A, et al. Effect of controlled volumetric tissue heating with radiofrequency on cellulite and the subcutaneous tissue of the buttocks and thighs. J Drugs Dermatol 2006;5(8):714–22.
27. Kaplan H, Gat A. Clinical and histopathological results following TriPollar radiofrequency skin treatments. J Cosmet Laser Ther 2009;11:78–84.
28. Manuskiatti W, Wachirakaphan C, Lektrakul N, Varothai S. Circumference reducation and cellulite treatment with a TriPollar radiofrequency device: a pilot study. JEADV 2009;23:820–7.
29. Krueger N, Levy H, Sadick NS. Safety and efficacy of a new device combining radiofrequency and low-frequency pulsed electromagnetic fields for the treatment of facial rhytides. J Drugs Dermatol 2012;11(11):1306–9.
30. Levy H. Evaluation of using Venus Freeze for skin tightening and cellulite treatment: study summary. Online. Available: <http://venusbackup.venustechnologies.info/wp-content/uploads/2013/08/Evaluation-of-Using-Venus-Freeze-Levy.pdf>.
31. Marini L. RF and pulsed magnetic field combination: an innovative approach to effectively addressing skin laxity, body reshaping, and cellulite. Presented at the Indonesian Society for

Aesthetic Medicine, Dec 2011, Jakarta, Indonesia. Online. Available: <http://www.glomedspa.com/images/stories/_2013_Venus_Freeze/Questions_and_Answers/RF_and_Pulsed_Magnetic_Field.pdf>.

32. Mulholland RS. Synergistic multi-polar radiofrequency and pulsed magnetic fields in the non-invasive treatment of skin laxity and body contouring. Online. Available: <http://venusbackup.venustechnologies.info/wp-content/uploads/2011/04/Dr.-Mulholland.pdf>.

33. Christ C, Brenke R, Sattler G, et al. Improvement in skin elasticity in the treatment of cellulite and connective tissue weakness by means of extracorporeal pulse activation therapy. Aesth Surg J 2008;28(5):538–44.

34. Adatto MA, Adatto-Neilson R, Novak P, et al. Body shaping with acoustic wave therapy AWT/EPAT: randomized, controlled study on 14 subjects. J Cosmet Laser Ther 2011;13:291–6.

35. Douer SZ, Feferberg IA. Bella contour medial study: a non-invasive medical device for: releasing body fat, breaking down cellulite, body contouring and sculpting. Online.

Available: <http://www.realaesthetics.com/images/stories/bellacontour/clinicstudies/bellacontour_medical_study_stevenZ.pdf>.

36. Rossi AM, Katz BE. A modern approach to the treatment of cellulite. Dermatol Clin 2014;32:51–9.

37. White WM, Makin IR, Slayton MH, et al. Selective transcutaneous delivery of energy to porcine soft tissues using intense ultrasound (IUS). Lasers Surg Med 2008;40:67–75.

38. White WM, Makin IR, Barthe PG, et al. Selective creation of thermal injury zones in the superficial musculoaponeurotic system using intense ultrasound therapy: a new target for noninvasive facial rejuvenation. Arch Facial Plast Surg 2007;9:22–9.

39. Alster TS, Tanzi EL. Noninvasive lifting of arm, thigh, and knee skin with transcutaneous intense focused ultrasound. Dermatol Surg 2012;38:754–9.

40. McKinney S. VASER Shape MC1 non-invasively reduces cellulite. The Aesthetic Guide 2010. Online. Available: <http://digital.miinews.com/article/VASER+Shape+MC1+Non-Invasively+Reduces+Cellulite/555581/53062/article.html>.

Subcision: Cellulite Reduction

16

Doris Hexsel, Camile L. Hexsel

Key Messages

- Subcision is a simple procedure to correct depressed cellulite lesions
- There is relationship between fibrous septa and depressed lesions, as shown in the literature
- Performed under local anesthesia, subcision is an outpatient procedure in which subcutaneous fibrous septa that pull the skin down are cut
- Good results are achieved with proper technique and when performed by experienced physicians
- The procedure is usually performed using a simple subcision needle and does not leave scars
- This procedure can be combined with other treatments for cellulite
- It can be repeated, if deemed necessary

Introduction

Originally described by Orentreich and Orentreich,[1] subcision ('subcutaneous incisionless surgery') is a very simple surgical technique for the treatment of wrinkles and scars on the face. In 1995, Hexsel and Mazzuco developed this technique for the specific treatment of cellulite.[2] In a study of 232 women with cellulite on the thighs and buttocks, 79% reported being satisfied with the improvement achieved in the first session of the procedure[3] with significant improvement and even the disappearance of depressed lesions in the treated areas.

In clinical practice, approximately 80% of patients undergoing subcision for the treatment of cellulite are found to be very satisfied with the results. The first author, who has the largest experience in the world in this technique, having treated approximately 2000 patients and who described the technique for the treatment of cellulite, considers subcision to have the advantage of being a simple, minimally invasive, low cost technique with immediate, reproducible and persistent results in the treatment of depressed lesions of cellulite, without the risk of scar formation or significant side effects. Moreover, this technique addresses the fibrous septa, which are responsible for the depressions of cellulite.[4]

Cellulite affects almost every woman. Although there are no precise data in different populations, prevalence higher than 90% is reported by different authors.[5] It most commonly affects thighs and buttocks, but it may also occur in the abdomen and arms. It is characterized by altered skin relief in the affected areas. Relative to the normal skin relief, the most common lesions are depressed which may alternate with raised areas.[6] Cellulite generally occurs after adolescence and tends to worsen with advancing age due to the superimposition of an aggravating factor: skin flaccidity. Another factor that aggravates this condition is the increased deposition of localized fat. Coincidentally, cellulite occurs in areas where a woman's body naturally stores fat.

Anatomic bases of the depressed lesions and action mechanism(s)

Over 30 years ago, Nürnberger and Müller[7] described the anatomical basis of cellulite, demonstrating the differences in the fat lobes of women and men that contribute to the predominant incidence and prevalence of this condition in women. Besides having a thicker layer of adipose tissue compared with men, women have larger and more rectangular fat lobes and perpendicular fibrous septa that attach the skin to the muscular fascia. These cause the projection of subcutaneous fat into the skin surface, thus causing the changes in relief typical of this condition: depressed lesions and raised areas. It is noteworthy that cellulite mainly occurs in the areas of fat deposition in women, such as the buttocks, thighs, and outer thighs. In those areas where fat is stored, cellulite is more difficult to eliminate by dieting, except through extreme diets that promote an intense weight loss.

In 2009, a study employing magnetic resonance imaging (MRI) showed the presence of thick subcutaneous septa in about 97% of the depressed lesions typical of cellulite, as evidence of its pathogenesis in this condition. These septa displayed a tree-like morphology. Furthermore, the T2 images also showed the presence of vessels together with the septa (Fig. 16.1).[4]

With the increased understanding of the pathogenesis and its relation to the most common feature seen in cellulite, the depressed lesions caused by a subcutaneous septa that pulls the skin down, subcision has become the procedure of choice for the treatment of depressed lesions

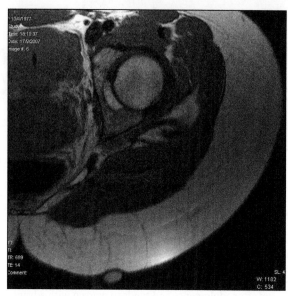

Figure 16.1 Magnetic resonance imaging of a depressed cellulite lesion with subjacent fibrous septa

of cellulite, by cutting those subcutaneous fibrous septa. It is an outpatient procedure performed under local anesthesia, and acts by three mechanisms of action:

- Sectioning of the subcutaneous fibrous septa, thus releasing the tension on the skin in the area of the depressed lesions[1]
- The formation of hematomas from sectioning of the accompanying vessel that is typically next to the subcutaneous septa, with subsequent fibroplasia, promoting a natural physiological filling of the lesions
- Redistribution of the traction forces produced by the subcutaneous septa and tension from the fat on the skin.[3]

Patient selection

Patients eligible for subcision are those with evident depressed lesions in the affected areas (thighs and buttocks) that are visible without the use of any maneuver, such as pinching the skin or muscle contraction.

Expectations should be realistic as there is no improvement in skin flaccidity or localized fat after subcision – conditions frequently seen in patients with depressed lesions. The bruises often produced by treatment may take 30–60 days to disappear and patients should be made aware of this. Failure to adhere to pre-operative instructions may result in cosmetic complications that are difficult to treat, such as iron deposition and discoloration resultant from it.

Contraindications to the procedure include the presence of coagulation disorders or the use of medications that interfere with local anesthetics or with the process of coagulation, systemic diseases, systemic or local active

infection, pregnancy, breastfeeding, and a history of keloids or hypertrophic scars.

As cellulite is a multifactorial condition, other measures are recommended to maintain the results including diet, exercise and weight control, among others.

Typical treatment course

Pre-operative instructions

Some instructions should be followed pre-operatively:

- Discontinue iron in medicines or food, for 1 month before the procedure.
- If possible, discontinue medications that interfere with blood coagulation, for 1–2 weeks before the procedure, such as nonsteroidal anti-inflammatory agents, ginkgo biloba, vitamin E and some hormones.
- Where present, treat possible local infections such as folliculitis.
- Do not undergo the procedure during the menstrual period.

Blood tests should be done 15 days before the procedure, including a coagulogram and other specific exams, according to the patient's history and needs. Pay special attention to potential thrombophilia candidates (history of thrombosis, abortion, etc.).

Day of the procedure

- As cellulite occurs in easily contaminated areas, the authors recommend the use of ciprofloxacin 500 mg twice a day for 3 days, starting 6 hours before the procedure. The authors also recommend acetaminophen 1 hour before and continued use, every 6 hours, for 2 days.
- Photographs are taken.
- A physical examination should be performed in the standing position with relaxed muscles and with illumination from above in order to better view and mark the lesions to be treated with a surgical pen.[3] It is recommended to select lesions 30 mm in diameter or smaller, or 30 mm portions of larger lesions,[2] to avoid formation of hematomas and dissection planes that are too large and can potentially lead to complications (Fig. 16.2).

Surgical procedure

- Antisepsis of the area with iodine alcohol or another antiseptic solution.
- A solution of 2% lidocaine with epinephrine diluted to 10–20% anesthetic solution with 0.9% saline comprising 80–90% of the volume is used, allowing more lesions to be treated than it would be possible if the anesthetic was more concentrated and not diluted. The authors recommend not exceeding a

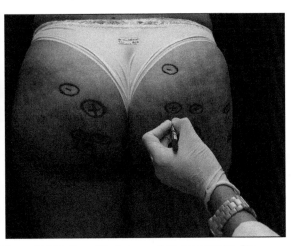

Figure 16.2 Marking of the lesions suitable for subcision. The symbols '+' highlight deeper lesions

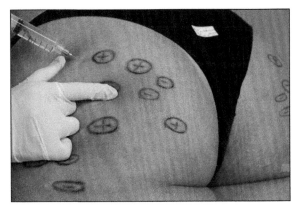

Figure 16.3 Local anesthesia is performed in the subcutaneous tissue level, under the lesion and beyond its borders. An anesthetic intradermal button 1–2 cm away from the lesion is prepared, where the subcision needle will be inserted

total dose greater than 7 mg of lidocaine per kg body weight. Tumescent anesthesia can also be used and it is very safe; however, this type of anesthesia tends to result in less hematoma formation. It should be pointed out that hematoma is desirable as it is described as one of the main mechanisms of action for subcision by Orentreich and Orentreich,[1] and subsequently by Hexsel and Mazzuco[2,3] for the treatment of cellulite.

- First, a focal superficial area of intradermal anesthesia is performed, with the goal of numbing the area where the long needle will be introduced for deeper subcutaneous anesthesia. This is done approximately 2 cm from the edges of the depressed lesion to be treated. Subsequently, local infiltrative anesthesia is performed in the subcutaneous plane where the incisions will be made, exceeding the limits of the depressed area to be treated. For this, a long thin needle is inserted to a depth from 1–2 cm beyond the edge of the marked lesion. The anesthetic is injected in a fanning pattern into the subcutaneous plane while withdrawing the needle (Fig. 16.3).

- Once the vasoconstrictor takes effect, when the skin becomes pale and there is evidence of piloerection, the tissue is pierced using an 18-gauge Nokor™ needle (BD) (Fig. 16.4A), introduced to a depth of 1.5 or 2 cm into the subcutaneous tissue and then directed parallel to the skin surface (Fig. 16.4B).

- The sectioning of the fibrous septa is achieved by pressing the needle against the septa while withdrawing the needle (Fig. 16.4C).

- Only those septa that exert traction on the skin should be sectioned, and the maintenance of some septa intact is recommended, especially in the lower buttocks and upper thighs, to avoid the risk of the occurrence of protrusion of subcutaneous fat as a complication.

- Once the septa have been sectioned, a slight pinch of the skin helps to determine the presence of residual septa exerting downward traction on the skin (Fig. 16.4D).

- With subcision, blood vessels accompanying the connective septa are also sectioned, immediately inducing bleeding and the consequent formation of hematomas. The amount of bleeding and the size of the hematoma can be controlled by compressing areas subjected to subcision for 5–10 minutes (normal clotting time) with a heavy pillow filled with sand and wrapped in sterile field or sterile pillow case (Fig. 16.5). This pillow weighs approximately 5 kg and ensures adequate hemostasis and control of the size of the hematomas.

The subcision is completed by cleaning the site and placing compressive dressings consisting of gauze and Micropore™ or paper tape (Fig. 16.6). Compressive clothing should be worn immediately following the surgical procedure.

Post-operative recommendations

The use of a prescribed antibiotic (ciprofloxacin) for 3 days is recommended. Analgesics may be prescribed. In general, if required, acetaminophen (500–1000 mg) every 6 hours is recommended. After 48–72 hours, the dressing should be removed. It is important that the patient wears compressive clothing during both night and day for 7 days and during the day for 30 days. Physical exercise should be suspended for 15 days and done only moderately in the first month.[8]

Other means of carrying out subcision

The use of a steel wire has been described as a method of performing the subcision procedure. The wire is inserted into the skin causing the sectioning of all the septa. This is a disadvantage because, in some areas, some septa need

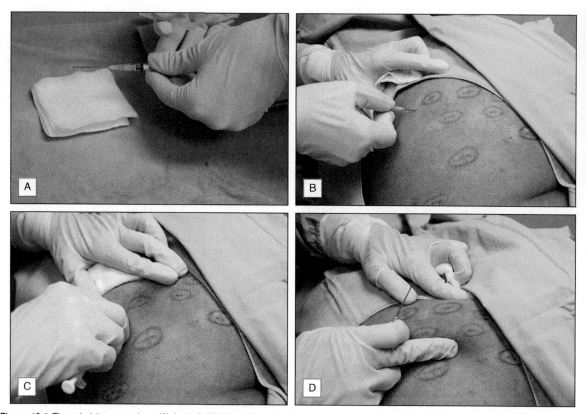

Figure 16.4 The subcision procedure. **(A)** An 18G BD Nokor™ needle is usually used to cut the septa. **(B)** The needle is inserted outside of the lesion, 1.5 or 2 cm into the subcutaneous tissue, and then parallel to the skin surface. **(C)** To sever the septa, the needle is pressed against it, while withdrawing the needle. **(D)** A slight pinch test is performed to check for residual septa pulling the skin down

to be preserved to avoid the complications mentioned above, such as herniation of fat, with the formation of large hematomas and/or areas of fibrosis in the areas subjected to the procedure.[9] Authors have reported different results using variations of the subcision technique. According to them, no significant benefits were found in patients with cellulite treated using subcision with steel wires and they also reported post-operative irregularities with this technique.[9]

The 1440 nm Nd:YAG (Cellulaze™, Cynosure, Chelmsford, MA) is a laser with a side-firing fiber and temperature-sensing cannula that induces rupture of subcutaneous septa from heat generated and induces the remodeling of the dermis and subcutaneous tissue. A study of the efficacy of treatment with 1440 nm pulsed Nd:YAG laser on grade II and III cellulite in 20 patients demonstrated, with objective measurements at 2 years, an increase over the baseline mean skin elasticity (34%) and mean dermal thickness (11%), and in the average percentage of dermal thickening determined by ultrasound imaging. Treatment efficacy was assessed by cellulite reduction by the Müller–Nürnberger scale. Most patients dropped to a lower severity level of cellulite within the same grade (II or III) but most did not change the grade of cellulite by that scale.[10] DiBernardo reported increase

in mean skin thickness (as shown by ultrasound) and skin elasticity after single treatment with a 1440 nm pulsed laser in 10 patients. Subjective physician evaluations indicated improvement in the appearance of cellulite.[11] In another study by DiBernardo and colleagues, 57 patients underwent one treatment with a 1440 nm Nd:YAG.[12] At 6 months post-treatment, blinded evaluators rated at least a 1-point improvement in the appearance of cellulite in 96% of treated sites, assessed using on a 5-point, 2-category ordinal photonumeric scale (number of evident dimples and severity of linear undulations/contour irregularities). Blinded evaluators correctly identified baseline versus post-treatment photos in 95% of cases.[12] Katz showed that blinded evaluators were able to identify baseline versus post-treatment two-dimensional photos in 90% of cases (one 1440 nm Nd:YAG treatment, 15 patients). Improvement in contour irregularities occurred in 94% of the sites. With three-dimensional, the average decrease in skin depressions was 49%, and 66% of patients showed improvement in overall skin contour at 6 months.[13]

Expected outcomes

Re-evaluations are recommended 30 and 60 days after the procedure, when complete regression of the hematomas

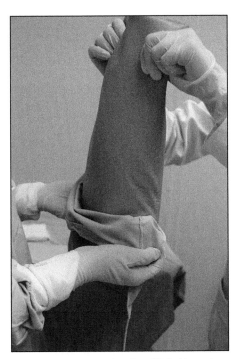

Figure 16.5 An approximately 5 kg pillow filled with sand wrapped in sterile fabric is used after sectioning the septa with subcision, to control bleeding and hematomas

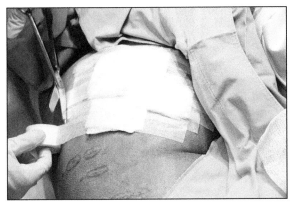

Figure 16.6 Compressive dressings after subcision, with gauze and Micropore™ paper tape, followed by compressive clothing

can be expected and the results evaluated, with visible improvement of the depressed lesions. If further subcision is indicated, it can be carried out when there are no apparent sequelae from the previous procedures, usually after 2–3 months.[14]

Safety, potential complications, and their prevention/management

Complications are usually rare and easy to manage when the proper technique is used by an experienced professional and the recommendations are followed by patients.

Bruising and ecchymosis, seroma and some local sensitivity are expected in this procedure and usually regress spontaneously.

Localized iron depositionto the skin/hemosiderosis with discoloration is a condition that can occur if patients fail to suspend the iron in food or medicines. It is difficult to treat, since it is a subcutaneous tattoo of the hematic pigment, hemosiderin. It should be prevented by making clear to the patient the importance of following the preoperative recommendations, especially in relation to the restriction of iron and the avoidance of undergoing the procedure during the menstrual period.

Sub-optimal response may occur in some lesions in which not all the septa responsible for depressed the skin are sectioned. In this case, the procedure may be repeated, as mentioned above.

Two complications are called 'excessive response' to subcision. The first, a true excessive response, is due to excessive fibroplasia. It might occur when large areas are subjected to subcision and when adequate care is not taken to control the size of the hematomas. It is easily treatable with local infiltration of triamcinolone in appropriate doses. The second, which is difficult to treat, arises from the sectioning of all the septa in certain areas or very superficial subcision, causing fat herniation and elevation of the treated area. It can be improved with localized liposuction and prolonged compression of the affected area.

Infection, erythema, edema, and contact dermatitis can also occur and are transitory. Hypertrophic and keloid scar formation and necrosis of the treated areas have not been reported.

CASE STUDY 1

A 29-year-old Caucasian woman with no significant present or past medical history came in for evaluation and treatment of cellulite. Medications include an oral contraceptive (drospirenone and ethinylestradiol). Her weight was 76.7 kg and 25.33 kg/m^2 of body mass index (BMI). The patient had depressed lesions on both sides of the thighs and buttocks, classified as severe cellulite by the new cellulite severity scale (CSS).[15] She underwent subcision in January 2014. Preoperative laboratory tests were normal. On the day of the procedure, the patient used a prophylactic antibiotic (ciprofloxacin 500 mg) and analgesic (acetaminophen 500 mg), taken for 3 and 2 days, respectively. The patient was instructed to wear compressive clothing in the treated areas for 30 days. The first evaluation was performed 4 days after the procedure, when the dressings were removed and the surgical area was examined. The second evaluation was 7 days after the procedure and the hematomas demonstrated excellent resolution. The third evaluation was performed 30 days after the procedure and a complete resolution of the hematomas was observed, as can be seen in Figure 16.7. Evaluations according to the CSS[15] showed grade 13 and 13 for the right and left buttocks respectively, before treatment, and decreased to grade 8 and 7 for right and left buttocks after the treatment.

Figure 16.7 A series of pictures of Patient #1. **(A)** Clinical appearance of cellulite before the procedure. **(B)** Hematomas 4 days after the procedure. **(C)** Hematomas 7 days after the procedure. **(D)** Clinical appearance 30 days after the procedure

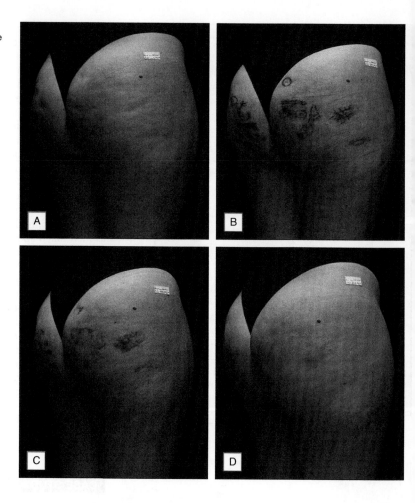

CASE STUDY 2

A 36-year-old Caucasian woman with no significant present or past medical history came in for evaluation and treatment of cellulite. Her weight was 77.5 kg and BMI was 26.02 kg/m². The patient had depressed lesions on both thighs and buttocks, classified as severe cellulite by the CSS.[15] Preoperative laboratory tests were normal. She had subcision in January 2014. Prophylactic antibiotics and pain control were the same as in Case 1, and she also used compressive clothing for 30 days after the procedure. The evaluations were performed 3, 7 and 30 days after the procedure with similar evolution, as can be observed in Figure 16.8. Evaluations according to the CSS[15] showed grade 14 and 13 for the right and left buttocks respectively, before treatment, and decreased to grade 9 and 9 for right and left buttocks after the treatment.

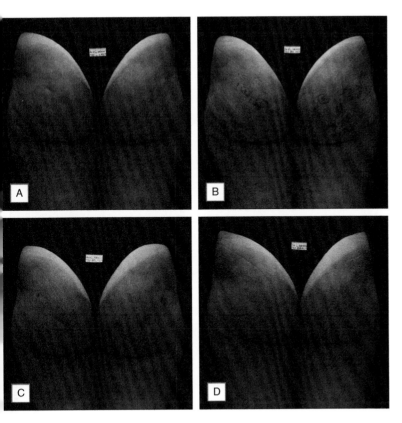

Figure 16.8 A series of pictures of Patient #2. **(A)** Clinical appearance of cellulite before the procedure. **(B)** Hematomas 3 days after the procedure. **(C)** Hematomas 7 days after the procedure. **(D)** Clinical appearance 30 days after the procedure

References

1. Orentreich DS, Orentreich N. Subcutaneous incisionless (subcision) surgery for the correction of depressed scars and wrinkles. Dermatol Surg 1995;21(6):543–9.
2. Hexsel DM, Mazzuco R. Subcision: uma alternativa cirúrgica para a lipodistrofia ginoide ('celulite') e outras alterações do relevo corporal. An Bras Dermatol 1997;72:27–32.
3. Hexsel DM, Mazzuco R. Subcision: a treatment for cellulite. Int J Dermatol 2000;39(7):539–44.
4. Hexsel DM, Abreu M, Rodrigues TC, et al. Side-by-side comparison of areas with and without cellulite depressions using magnetic resonance imaging. Dermatol Surg 2009;35(10):1471–7.
5. Avram MM. Cellulite: a review of its physiology and treatment. J Cosmet Laser Ther 2004;6(4):181–5.
6. Draelos ZD. Cellulite. Etiology and purported treatment. Dermatol Surg 1997;23:1177–81.
7. Nürnberger F, Müller G. So-called cellulite: an invented disease. J Dermatol Surg Oncol 1978;4(3):221–9.
8. Hexsel DM, Soirefmann M, Dal'Forno T. Subcision for cellulite. In: Katz B, Sadick NS, editors. Procedures in cosmetic dermatology: body contouring. Saunders Elsevier; 2010. p. 157–64.
9. Sasaki GH. Comparison of results of wire subcision performed alone, with fills, and/or with adjacent surgical procedures. Aesthet Surg J 2008;28(6):619–26.
10. Sasaki GH. Single treatment of grades II and III cellulite using a minimally invasive 1,440-nm pulsed Nd:YAG laser and side-firing fiber: an institutional review board-approved study with a 24-month follow-up period. Aesthetic Plast Surg 2013;37(6):1073–89.
11. DiBernardo BE. Treatment of cellulite using a 1440-nm pulsed laser with one-year follow-up. Aesthet Surg J 2011;31(3):328–41.
12. DiBernardo B, Sasaki G, Katz BE, et al. A multicenter study for a single, three-step laser treatment for cellulite using a 1440-nm Nd:YAG laser, a novel side-firing fiber, and a temperature-sensing cannula. Aesthet Surg J 2013;33(4):576–84.
13. Katz B. Quantitative & qualitative evaluation of the efficacy of a 1440 nm Nd:YAG laser with novel bi-directional optical fiber in the treatment of cellulite as measured by 3-dimensional surface imaging. J Drugs Dermatol 2013;12(11):1224–30.
14. Hexsel D, Mazzuco R, Soirefmann M. Subcision. In: Goldman M, Hexsel D, editors. Cellulite: pathophysiology and treatment. 2nd ed. London: Informa Health Care; 2010. p. 174–9.
15. Hexsel DM, Hexsel CL, Dal'Forno T. A validated photonumeric cellulite severity scale. J Eur Acad Dermatol Venereol 2009;23(5):523–8.

Page numbers followed by "f" indicate figures, "t" indicate tables, and "b" indicate boxes.

Printed and bound by CPI Group (UK) Ltd, Croydon, CR0 4YY

08/05/2025

01864756-0001